ACUTE LUNG INJURY: FROM INFLAMMATION TO REPAIR

Biomedical and Health Research

Volume 34

Earlier published in this series

ISSN: 0929-6743

UCL Molecular Pathology series

Editor: D.S. Latchman

From Genetics to Gene Therapy
Autoimmune Diseases: Focus on Sjögren's Syndrome
Apoptosis and Cell Cycle Control in Cancer
Ischaemia: Preconditioning and Adaptation
Genetics of Common Diseases: Future Therapeutic and Diagnostic Possibilities
A Molecular Approach to Parkinson's Disease

Acute Lung Injury:
From Inflammation to Repair

Edited by

Geoffrey J. Bellingan

Centre for Cardiopulmonary Biochemistry & Respiratory Medicine,
Royal Free and University College Medical School
Rayne Institute, London, United Kingdom

and

Geoffrey J. Laurent

Centre for Cardiopulmonary Biochemistry & Respiratory Medicine,
Royal Free and University College Medical School
Rayne Institute, London, United Kingdom

IOS
Press

Ohmsha

Amsterdam • Berlin • Oxford • Tokyo • Washington, DC

BS

ISBN 90 5199 503 2 (IOS Press)
ISBN 4 274 90355 9 C3047 (Ohmsha)
Library of Congress Catalog Card Number: 00-101364

Publisher
IOS Press
Van Diemenstraat 94
1013 CN Amsterdam
The Netherlands
fax: +31 20 620 3419
e-mail: order@iospress.nl

Distributor in the UK and Ireland
IOS Press/Lavis Marketing
73 Lime Walk
Headington
Oxford OX3 7AD
England
fax: +44 1865 75 0079

Distributor in the USA and Canada
IOS Press, Inc.
5795-G Burke Centre Parkway
Burke, VA 22015
USA
fax: +1 703 323 3668
e-mail: iosbooks@iospress.com

Distributor in Germany
IOS Press
Spandauer Strasse 2
D-10178 Berlin
Germany
fax: +49 30 242 3113

Distributor in Japan
Ohmsha, Ltd.
3-1 Kanda Nishiki-cho
Chiyoda-ku, Tokyo 101
Japan
fax: +81 3 3233 2426

PRINTED IN THE NETHERLANDS

3/20/03

List of Contributors

Geoffrey J. Bellingan
Centre for Cardiopulmonary Biochemistry & Respiratory Medicine
Royal Free and University College Medical School
Rayne Institute
London UK

Richard Bucala
The Picower Institute for Medical Research
Manhasset
New York NY 11030 USA

Rachel C Chambers
Centre for Cardiopulmonary Biochemistry & Respiratory Medicine
Royal Free University College Medical School
Rayne Institute
University Street
London UK

Seamus C. Donnelly
Rayne Laboratory
Respiratory Medicine Unit
University of Edinburgh
Teviot Place
Edinburgh Scotland

Mark Griffiths
Adult Intensive Care Unit
Royal Brompton Hospital
Sydney Street
London UK

Nick Hirani
Rayne Laboratory
Respiratory Medicine Unit
University of Edinburgh
Teviot Place
Edinburgh Scotland

Gerard F. Hoyne
Respiratory Medicine Unit
University of Edinburgh Medical School
Teviot Place
Edinburgh Scotland

Geoffrey J. Laurent
Centre for Cardiopulmonary Biochemistry & Respiratory Medicine
Royal Free and University College Medical School
Rayne Institute
London UK

William MacNee
Medical & Radiological Sciences
ELEGI, Colt Research Laboratories,
Wilkie Building
University of Edinburgh
Edinburgh Scotland

Richard P. Marshall
Centre for Cardiopulmonary Biochemistry & Respiratory Medicine
Royal Free University College Medical School
Rayne Institute
University Street
London UK

Antonia Orsi
Wolfson Institute for Biomedical Research
University College Medical School
London UK

Daryl D. Rees
Phytopharm Plc
Godmanchester
Cambs. UK

Robert A. Stockley
Department of Medicine
Queen Elizabeth Hospital
Birmingham UK

Terry D. Tetley
Department of Respiratory Medicine
Charing Cross Hospital
Imperial College School of Medicine
London UK

Contents

Acute Lung Injury: From Inflammation to Repair
G.J. Bellingan and G.J. Laurent (Eds.)
IOS Press, 2000

An Introduction to Acute Lung Injury

Geoffrey J. Bellingan and Geoffrey J. Laurent

Centre for Cardiopulmonary Biochemistry & Respiratory Medicine
Royal Free and University College Medical School
London, UK

1   Acute lung injury - a success story.

The treatment of acute lung injury (ALI) and the most severe form of this condition namely the Acute Respiratory Distress Syndrome (ARDS) is one of the success stories of the last decade. The mortality of ARDS has fallen dramatically from 70 - 90% in the 1970s to 30 - 50% over the last few years [1-3]. The reasons for this improvement are many but include a greater understanding of the condition in addition to a multitude of practical improvements in clinical intensive care. Despite this better understanding and the improving survival figures there is much that we do not know about the molecular mechanisms underlying acute lung injury. This book focuses on important recent advances in cellular and molecular pathology of inflammation and repair as they apply to respiratory medicine, presenting an in-depth approach covering those areas where progress has been most rapid. As inflammation and repair mechanisms are central to such a wide range of pulmonary pathology the chapters have been designed not to focus simply on acute lung injury and ARDS but to examine common ground between ARDS, asthma, chronic obstructive pulmonary disease and the fields of allergy/immunology and sepsis. This book forms part of a highly successful series of molecular pathology symposia that have been run by Professor Latchman at the Windeyer Institute of Medical Sciences, University College London over the past seven years. Twelve international experts, chosen to provide a broad approach covering all the essential topics in molecular aspects of pulmonary disease, were invited to address the conference. This volume is derived from the contributions of many of these speakers with additional chapters provided by other experts in this rapidly advancing field.

In the first section this book examines mechanisms of inflammation and repair, with a broad introduction to these process followed by chapters specifically focusing on molecules, cytokines and cells of interest. Daryl Rees and Antonia Orsi provide an excellent review of the multitude of roles on nitric oxide (NO) in inflammation leading up to developments at the cutting edge of this field while Seamus Donnelly, Nick Hirani and Rick Bucala outline the role of macrophage migration inhibition factor (MIF) in inflammation and provide evidence to support the rationale for an anti-MIF therapeutic strategy. Bill McNee's authoritative chapter on oxidative stress in lung injury illustrates clearly the detailed understanding we now have of this field while Rob Stockley describes significant recent advances in the understanding of the role of neutrophils both in lung defence and as effector cells in lung damage. A novel approach to therapy is then provided by Gerard Hoyne who discusses the potential for reduction of inflammation by the induction of tolerance. Finally in the section on inflammation Mark Griffith covers the key subject of transgenic and knockout mice and their use — current and future — in the investigation of the pathogenesis of pulmonary inflammation.

It has become increasingly clear that repair mechanisms are not only essential to the appropriate resolution of lung injury but that like inflammatory mechanisms these too can lead to severe consequences when inappropriately regulated. The second section of this book provides an informative update on mechanisms of repair with a chapter by Terry Tetley covering key developments in the protease-antiprotease story in ALI as well as chapters on novel pro-fibrotic molecules and mechanisms by Rachel Chambers, Richard Marshall and ourselves. Overall readers should gain an excellent insight into new developments in molecular aspects of this exciting area of medicine. First however it is important to put these cellular and molecular discoveries into context. What is ALI, how important is it, how does it arise, what is the outcome and how do the topics covered in this book translate into the clinical arena?

2   What is acute lung injury?

This is a condition characterised by tachypnoea, severe hypoxaemia and diffuse bilateral pulmonary infiltrates arising as a consequence of an acute insult. The clinical aspects of this condition including definition, performance, clinical therapy and clinical trials have been recently reviewed [4-7]. The definitions of ALI and ARDS are shown in Table 1.

Table 1.
Consensus criteria for ARDS, (Bernard et al 1994).

	Acute lung injury	**ARDS**
Timing	acute onset	
Oxygenation	$PaO_2/FiO_2 < 40$ kPa[1] regardless of PEEP[2]	$PaO_2/FiO_2 < 26.6$ kPa[1] regardless of PEEP[2]
X ray	bilateral infiltrates on frontal chest X-ray	
PAWP[3]	<18mmHg with no evidence of left atrial hypertension	

[1]PaO_2/FiO_2 ratio is the arterial partial pressure of oxygen divided by the fractional inspired oxygen.

[2]Positive end expiratory pressure (PEEP) is set on a mechanical ventilator.

[3]PAWP - pulmonary artery wedge pressure.

Notes:
- Mechanical ventilation is not a requirement for these definitions.
- ALI and ARDS are not specific diseases rather syndromes arising from inflammation and increased permeability.
- The onset should be acute to exclude chronic lung disease but there were no specific recommendations as to the exact time frame for the term acute.

A wide range of initiating injuries have been described but all lead to increased capillary permeability, usually occurring as part of a systemic inflammatory response. Although ALI is recognised as a common and serious problem with a high mortality and significant impact both in terms of morbidity and cost of care, there is lack of clarity as to its definition and incidence. The American-European consensus conference on acute respiratory distress syndrome (ARDS) recognised that the definition of ARDS as a condition would entail arbitrary cut-off points for blood gas and chest x-ray abnormalities [8]. In light of this they adopted the term ALI to apply to the spectrum of this "continuum of pathologic processes" and reserved the term ARDS for the most severe end of this spectrum. Despite their many recognised drawbacks the current definitions are clear and simple and have now allowed excellent demographic studies of ALI and ARDS and have focused clinical and basic research more clearly than before. It remains important however to remember that despite such simple definitions the conditions are still remarkably heterogeneous and this heterogeneity can lead to many problems with studies both of underlying disease mechanisms and of novel therapies. The initiating insult can be either directly to the lungs or indirectly to a distant part of the body with sepsis, trauma and gastric aspiration accounting for more than three quarters of cases; some of the causes of ALI are listed in Table 2 [9, 10].

Table 2.
A list of some of the causes of ALI/ARDS.

Intrathoracic	Extrathoracic
Aspiration of gastric contents	Sepsis
Smoke inhalation	Multiple trauma
Near Drowning	Acute pancreatitis
Pulmonary emboli	Massive Transfusion
	Burns
	Head injury

3   How important is acute lung injury?

Through these definitions we now have a much clearer idea of the incidence of ALI and ARDS. For example estimates for the incidence of ALI in USA in the 1970's were in the order of 70+ patients per 100,000 residents per year but now more realistic estimates are available [11]. In a prospective study of all 13,346 admissions (>15 years) over an 8 week period undertaken in Sweden, Denmark and Iceland Luhr et al. identified 287 ALI and 221 ARDS patients [12]. This gives an incidence of 17.9 for ALI per 100,000 and 13.5 for ARDS per 100,000 population per year. Another recent study from Finland indicated an incidence of 4.9 cases of ARDS per 100,000 inhabitants per year while Webster et al. suggested an incidence of 4.5 cases per 100,000 resident in the UK in 1985 [3, 13]. Another feature arising from the consensus definitions was that they led to clearer demographic studies and these demonstrated that the artificial PaO_2/FiO_2 cut-off of 27kPa (200 mmHg) for ARDS did not necessarily distinguish a sicker cohort of patients [8, 11]. This highlights that the simple definitions do not describe a defined patient group and that many factors including initiating insult, premorbid condition, age, speed of onset of other organ failures and many more all contribute to outcome. As highlighted earlier the mortality rate from ARDS was extraordinarily high in the 1970's with large series reporting mortalities of over 90% [14]. This has fallen steadily but still remains high at between 30 and 50% [3, 15]. Death is commonly from sepsis or SIRS, rather than from intractable hypoxaemia [16]. Along with sepsis other poor prognostic factors include early non-pulmonary organ failure, and chronic liver disease [11]. Survivors of ARDS as a group have worse outcome indices than other ICU cohorts admitted with similar injury severity and this is mainly due to persisting respiratory dysfunction [17]. Furthermore the care of patients with ARDS is usually protracted and always demanding. A recent estimate suggests that the costs of intensive care alone per survivor are over £ 44,000 (US $ 73,000) [3]. Thus ARDS is still a devastating condition which remains a huge human and financial burden.

4   How does acute lung injury arise?

ALI is clearly recognised to be a syndrome of inflammation and increased permeability, but despite considerable effort the American-European consensus committee could not reach agreement on the order of event in the pathogenesis of the lung injury [8]. Typically ARDS is described as having three phases, an exudative phase followed by a proliferative phase and finally a fibrotic phase [18-20]. These pathological descriptions are dogged by numerous difficulties including lack of biopsy samples, the effects of ventilator-induced injury, intercurrent nosocomial pneumonia and selection bias with most studies using post mortem tissue. As discussed in chapter 9 the timing of these stages are now more open to question, especially as to the initiation of fibroproliferative repair mechanisms. Aggressive inflammation and capillary leak are however key early events and the molecular aspects of this will be reviewed in chapter 2.

5   How do the topics covered in this book translate into the clinical arena?

The mortality from ARDS is falling steadily. The reasons for this are complex but include a better understanding of mechanisms driving the inflammatory response. It is now clear that mechanical ventilation itself can damage the lung, with over-distension of the lung leading to a damaging pro-inflammatory response and that responding by limiting tidal volumes in these patients has had a significant effect on outcome [21, 22]. Other advances include the correct timing of the use of steroids in ARDS. It has been recognised for some time that steroids can be detrimental early in ARDS but our greater understanding of the processes of inflammation and repair has led to the reintroduction of steroids as a late rescue therapy for fibrosis in ARDS [20, 23, 24]. These are two examples of how basic scientific advances and clinical improvement go hand in hand. Another area where science has moved from the bench to the bedside is in trials of biological mediators and their inhibitors. For example, there are currently multinational trials of antiprotease and surfactant therapy underway in ARDS. There have however been many failures in the use of biological therapies and it is important that lessons are learned from these. One key reason for failure was the inappropriate choice of animal models. The development of appropriate models will be a vital element of future scientific endeavour and is addressed in chapter 8. Another problem has been an incomplete understanding of the inflammatory and repair mechanisms, again highlighting the importance of basic scientific understanding to advances in the clinical arena.

6   What is the outcome of acute lung injury?

As already discussed the mortality form ARDS has improved dramatically, what however is the functional outcome of the survivors? There has been far less research in this direction and studies are difficult to perform and interpret due to numerous confounding variables. Despite this several interesting features are becoming apparent. Pulmonary function studies in survivors suggest that lung mechanics as a rule return to base line but that this recovery may be delayed for up to a year [11, 18, 25, 26]. There are however a number of survivors in whom gas exchange abnormalities persist with findings of increased dead space on exercise, low diffusion capacity and in those with abnormalities pulmonary artery pressures may be elevated [18]. These findings are not consistent but results suggest that there is a correlation between severity of ARDS and later pulmonary function abnormalities. Thus although the mortality of this condition has improved it still remains unacceptably high and there is also much room for improvement in functional outcome of survivors.

References.

1.   Milberg JA, Davis DR, Steinberg KP, Hudson LD (1995) Improved survival of patients with acute respiratory distress syndrome (ARDS): 1983-1993. *JAMA* **273:** 306-9
2.   Abel SJ, Finney SJ, Brett SJ, Keogh BF, Morgan CJ, Evans TW (1998) Reduced mortality in association with the acute respiratory distress syndrome (ARDS). *Thorax* **53:** 292-4
3.   Valta P, Uusaro A, Nunes S, Ruokonen E, Takala J (1999) Acute respiratory distress syndrome: frequency, clinical course, and costs of care. *Crit. Care Med.* **27:** 2367-74
4.   Lewandowski K (1999) Epidemiological data challenge ARDS/ALI definition. *Intensive Care Med.* **25:** 884-6
5.   Steltzer H, Krafft P (1999) Improved outcome of ARDS patients: are we really performing better? *Intensive Care Med.* **25:** 887-9
6.   Brochard L, Lemaire F (1999) Tidal volume, positive end-expiratory pressure, and mortality in acute respiratory distress syndrome. *Crit. Care Med.* **27:** 1661-3
7.   Brochard L, Brun-Buisson C (1999) Clinical trials in acute respiratory distress syndrome: what is ARDS? *Crit. Care Med.* **27:** 1657-8
8.   Bernard GR, Artigas A, Brigham KL, Carlet J, Falke K, Hudson L, Lamy M, Legall JR, Morris A, Spragg R (1994) The American-European Consensus Conference on ARDS. Definitions, mechanisms, relevant outcomes, and clinical trial co-ordination. *Am. J. Respir. Crit. Care Med.* **149:** 818-24
9.   Hudson LD, Milberg JA, Anardi D, Maunder RJ (1995) Clinical risks for development of the acute respiratory distress syndrome. *Am. J. Respir. Crit. Care Med.* **151:** 293-301
10.   G. Deby-Dupont M. Lamy (1999) Pathophysiology of acute respiratory distress syndrome and acute lung injury. *In* Oxford Textbook of Critical Care. *Eds.* A. Webb MJ. Shapiro M. Singer and PM. Suter. Oxford University Press. Oxford p 55-59
11.   Luce JM (1998) Acute lung injury and the acute respiratory distress syndrome. *Crit. Care Med.* **26:** 369-76
12.   Luhr OR, Antonsen K, Karlsson M, Aardal S, Thorsteinsson A, Frostell CG, Bonde J (1999) Incidence and mortality after acute respiratory failure and acute respiratory distress syndrome in Sweden, Denmark, and Iceland. The ARF Study Group. *Am. J. Respir. Crit. Care Med.* **159:** 1849-61
13.   Webster NR, Cohen AT, Nunn JF (1988) Adult respiratory distress syndrome--how many cases in the UK? *Anaesthesia* **43:** 923-6
14.   Zapol WM, Snider MT, Hill JD, Fallat RJ, Bartlett RH, Edmunds LH, Morris AH, Peirce EC 2d, Thomas AN, Proctor HJ, Drinker PA, Pratt PC, Bagniewski A, Miller RG Jr (1979) Extracorporeal membrane oxygenation in severe acute respiratory failure. A randomised prospective study. *JAMA* **242:** 2193-6
15.   Peek GJ, Moore HM, Moore N, Sosnowski AW, Firmin RK (1997) Extracorporeal membrane oxygenation for adult respiratory failure. *Chest* **112:** 759-64
16.   Montgomery AB, Stager MA, Carrico CJ, Hudson LD (1985) Causes of mortality in patients with the adult respiratory distress syndrome. *Am. Rev. Respir. Dis.* **132:** 485-9
17.   Davidson TA, Caldwell ES, Curtis JR, Hudson LD, Steinberg KP (1999) Reduced quality of life in survivors of acute respiratory distress syndrome compared with critically ill control patients. *JAMA* **281:** 354-60
18.   Griffiths MJD and Evans TW (1995) Adult respiratory distress syndrome. *In* Respiratory Medicine (2nd Ed) Eds. Brewis RAL, Corrin, B Geddes DM and Gibson GJ. W.B. Saunders Press p605-629
19.   Marshall R, Bellingan G, Laurent G (1998) The acute respiratory distress syndrome: fibrosis in the fast lane. *Thorax* **53:** 815-7
20.   Bellingan G (1999) Steroids in ARDS. *In:* Critical Care Focus. Ed Galley H. BMJ Press p 37-51
21.   National Institutes of health (NIH), National Heart, Lung and Blood Institutes news a and press releases web site: http://www.nhlbi.nih.gov/new/press/hlbi15-9.htm

22.   Ranieri VM, Suter PM, Tortorella C, De Tullio R, Dayer JM, Brienza A, Bruno F, Slutsky AS (1999) Effect of mechanical ventilation on inflammatory mediators in patients with acute respiratory distress syndrome: a randomised controlled trial. *JAMA* **282:** 54-61
23.   Bernard GR, Luce JM, Sprung CL, Rinaldo JE, Tate RM, Sibbald WJ, Kariman K, Higgins S, Bradley R, Metz CA, et al (1987) High-dose corticosteroids in patients with the adult respiratory distress syndrome. *N. Engl. J. Med.* **317:** 1565-70
24.   Meduri GU, Headley AS, Golden E, Carson SJ, Umberger RA, Kelso T, Tolley EA (1998) Effect of prolonged methylprednisolone therapy in unresolving acute respiratory distress syndrome: a randomised controlled trial. *JAMA* **280:** 159-65
25.   McHugh LG, Milberg JA, Whitcomb ME, Schoene RB, Maunder RJ, Hudson LD (1994) Recovery of function in survivors of the acute respiratory distress syndrome. *Am. J. Respir. Crit. Care Med.* **150:** 90-4
26.   Davidson TA, Rubenfeld GD, Caldwell ES, Hudson LD, Steinberg KP (1999) The Effect of Acute Respiratory Distress Syndrome on Long-term Survival. *Am J Respir Crit. Care Med.* **160:** 1838-1842

Acute Lung Injury: From Inflammation to Repair
G.J. Bellingan and G.J. Laurent (Eds.)
IOS Press, 2000

Mechanisms of Inflammation

Geoffrey J. Bellingan

Centre for Cardiopulmonary Biochemistry & Respiratory Medicine
Royal Free and University College Medical School
London, UK

Our understanding of the cellular and molecular processes in inflammation have advanced enormously over the last few decades. There are now detailed descriptions of the adhesion molecule families, chemokines and cytokines, the fundamental importance of matrix-cell interactions, free radical biology, including the explosion of work on nitric oxide and its synthetic pathways and the protease-anti-protease systems. This is in addition to advances made in the understanding of other regulatory cascades including the coagulation, complement and renin-angiotensin systems. There is also a wealth of new information on the molecular mechanisms through which pathogenic organisms cause disease in man, epitomised by the fascinating story for endotoxin, with its interaction with lipopolysaccharide binding protein and CD14 and the elucidation of the Toll-like receptors as their signal transduction system. Overlying all of these advances are novel discoveries on the genetics of the inflammatory response. This chapter will review our understanding of inflammation in relation to the pathogenesis of ALI so that the ensuing chapters on recent developments can be put into a broader context.

1   Definitions.

The most common agents initiating inflammation are bacterial cell wall components including lipopolysaccharide (LPS) from Gram-negative bacteria and teichoic acid and peptidoglycans from Gram-positive bacteria [1]. Other conditions however such as multiple trauma and pancreatitis also result in generalised inflammation in the absence of infection. With local inflammation both infective and non-infective insults commonly yield a similar clinical picture with the classic clinical findings of *calor, rubor, tumor and dolor.* When there is a systemic response to infective and non-infective insults the clinical condition is now referred to as the systemic inflammatory response syndrome (SIRS) [2, 3]. This is a multi-system inflammatory state characterised by excessive immuno-inflammatory cascade activation which can progress to a widespread reduction in cellular oxygen utilisation, ATP depletion, cell injury and death. The clinical features of SIRS are listed in Table 1. Acute lung injury is typically seen as part of SIRS although it can occur as an isolated organ failure or part of a multi-organ dysfunction syndrome (MODS) [4,5].

Table 1.
Criteria for the diagnosis of the systemic inflammatory response syndrome:

A severe clinical illness with the presence of two or more of the following criteria:
Temperature *(>38°c or <36°c)*
Tachycardia *(>90 beats/min)*
Tachypnoea *(respiratory rate >20 breaths/min or PaCO$_2$<4.25kPa (32mmHg)*
Altered white blood cell count *(>12 x 109/l or <4 x 109/l or more than 10% band forms on the peripheral blood film)*

Sepsis is the term used when SIRS is caused by documented infection.
In those patients in whom infection has led to organ dysfunction and hypotension the additional terms severe sepsis and septic shock are used.
Severe sepsis requires the presence of hypotension (systolic blood pressure of <90 mmHg or a drop of more than 40 mmHg from baseline) and one or more of the following as evidence of organ dysfunction in the absence of another obvious explanation other than sepsis:

- Metabolic acidosis.
- Arterial hypoxaemia (PaO$_2$<9.75 kPa (75 mmHg) or PaO$_2$/FiO$_2$ ratio of < 33.3 kPa (250 mmHg)).
- Oliguria (<0.03L/h for 3 hours or 0.7L/h for 24 hours).
- Coagulopathy (increase in prothrombin time of 50% or more or drop in platelet count of 50% or more or to <100 x 10^9/l).
- Encephalopathy (Glasgow coma score <14).

Septic shock is defined as hypotension persisting for more than 1 hour despite administration of adequate fluid for intravascular volume expansion, associated with signs of organ dysfunction.

2   Initiation and regulation of inflammation.

2.1   Cells involved in the inflammatory process.

Inflammation is a highly complex and integrated system in which the key players are the inflammatory cells and multiple mediator networks [6-8]. Inflammatory cells include the neutrophils, the monocyte-macrophage series, eosinophils, mast cells and cells of the immune system including T and B lymphocytes and dendritic cells. Neutrophils and macrophages are central to the inflammatory processes as they phagocytose and kill invading pathogens and are powerful regulators of local and systemic inflammatory responses through elaboration and secretion of a range of powerful mediators including cytokines, chemokines, growth factors, enzymes, lipid mediators and free radicals. The phagocytes contribute to innate immunity and through specific mediator signals interact with the lymphocytes invoking a powerful adaptive immune response. It must be remembered that a range of other cells including endothelial cells, mesothelial cells and fibroblasts can also elaborate pro-inflammatory cytokines and chemokines, produce free radicals phagocytose apoptotic cells and even present antigen [7]. These cells are also fundamentally important in regulating the inflammatory response and play particularly important roles in wound healing and tissue repair. For example in the lung fibroblasts along with endothelial and epithelial cells can reproduce much of the classic inflammatory response including elaboration of cytokines such as IL-1 and TGF-β which are directly implicated in the pathogenesis of ARDS and consequent fibrosis [9-11]. Hence a greater understanding of the involvement of stromal cells in the inflammatory response is required especially in regard to inflammation limited to specific regions/organs.

2.2   Priming and activation.

Normally inflammatory cells exist in a resting state and require specific signals for activation [12]. Activation is usually divided into two stages, priming and activation where priming is defined as a process whereby the response of an inflammatory cell to an activating stimulus is significantly potentiated by prior exposure to a priming agent.

Endotoxin or lipopolysaccharide (LPS) is the most widely known activating agent. It is a key component of the cell wall of Gram-negative bacteria. The major cell receptor for LPS is CD14 and this employs the Toll-like receptors for signal transduction [13, 14]. Other bacterial agents for example lipoteicoic acid, the peptidoglycans and N-formyl-L-methionyl-L-leucyl-phenylalanine (fMLP) from Gram-positive bacteria are also powerful activating agents with their own distinct receptor populations [15]. In addition to bacterial products, numerous endogenous agents such as pro-inflammatory cytokines can act as activators of inflammatory cells. The archetypal pro-inflammatory cytokines are tumour necrosis factor-α (TNF-α), interleukin-1β (IL-1β) and interleukin-6 (IL-6). TNF-α is rapidly detectable after a bacterial challenge, followed within a matter of hours by IL-1 and then IL-6. Other cytokines detectable after endotoxin challenge include IL-8, MIP-1α and MCP-1 [16]. TNF-α in particular, but also IL-1, is responsible for the release of these other cytokines. In animal models of sepsis or endotoxaemia neutralising antibodies to TNF-α abolishes the release of these later cytokines [17]. IL-6 stimulates acute phase protein production. In BAL fluid from ARDS patients the net pro-inflammatory capacity has been attributed to IL-1 not TNF-α [18]. Numerous cytokines have been detected in patients with acute lung injury as shown in Table 2

Table 2.
Cytokines detected in BAL fluid of patients with acute lung injury.

Tumour Necrosis Factor-α
Interleukin-1β,
Interluekin-2
Interluekin-4
Interluekin-6
Interluekin-8
Transforming Growth Factor-β
Insulin-like Growth Factor-1
Platelet Derived Growth Factor (like)
Transforming Growth Factor-α
Hepatocyte growth

Activation responses are embodied by enhanced microbicidal functional capacity, such as up-regulation of adhesion molecule expression and function, increased phagocytosis and enhanced superoxide production [6]. Activating signals not only boost inflammatory cell function but increase their numbers, promoting recruitment of marginating pools of leukocytes, enhanced release of precursors from the bone marrow and prolonging the life-span of inflammatory cells. Many priming and activating agents are also powerful chemotactic agents. BAL fluid of patients with ARDS has high levels of chemotactic activity, much of which cannot be explained by the classic chemotactic agents,

C5a and leukotriene B4. IL-8 is a potent neutrophil chemotactic agent and this is increased in the BAL of patients who develop ARDS. Indeed it is a powerful prognostic factor in predicting the development of ARDS in those at risk of this condition [19]. There is now evidence that IL-8 gene expression may be further regulated by periods of hypoxia/hyperoxia [20].

Extravasation of leukocytes from the blood stream into sites of inflammation requires both a chemotactic gradient and co-ordinated up-regulation of endothelial and inflammatory cell adhesion molecule expression. E and P-selectins are rapidly up-regulated on the endothelial surface and these, along with L-selectin, mediate leukocyte rolling, a process that slows leukocyte passage and allows for firm adhesion and transmigration. The β_2 integrins LFA-1 (CD11a), Mac-1 (CD11b) and p150/95 (CD11c) are the main leukocyte adhesion molecules responsible for firm adhesion, their endothelial ligands are ICAM-1 (CD54), ICAM-2 (CD102) and VCAM-1 (CD106). PECAM (CD31) and VLA-4 (CD29/CD49d) are essential for transmigration. Integrins are not simply involved with leukocyte adhesion and transmigration [21]. Knockout mice deficient in the $\beta 6$ integrin have increased numbers of pulmonary leukocytes and this phenotype is suppressed by $\alpha v \beta 6$ expression [22]. Interestingly these mice are protected from bleomycin induced fibrosis, a situation of enhanced inflammation but protection from fibrosis. A similar finding occurs in TGF-β knockout mice [23].

2.3   Aggressive inflammation SIRS and ARDS.

The inflammatory response can not only protect the body from the threat of invasion but, when inappropriately or excessively activated, can damage to the host itself as discussed with SIRS. More than 25 years ago Lewis Thomas eloquently described the potential of leukocytes to "overreact" and damage the host. He wrote "It is the information carried by the bacteria that we cannot abide. The Gram-negative bacteria are the best examples of this. They display lipopolysaccharide endotoxin in their walls, and these macromolecules are read by our tissues as the very worst of bad news. When we sense lipopolysaccharide, we are likely to turn on every defence at our disposal" [24]. There are now a large number of studies demonstrating the potential for leukocytes to damage host tissues and the ability of leukocyte depletion to protect in a range of inflammatory models.

Table 3.
Situations in which leukocyte depletion is beneficial.

Inflammatory models benefited by leukocyte depletion
Acute lung injury
Ischaemia reperfusion injuries:
Cardiac surgery
Compartment syndrome
Pancreatitis
Ischaemic Colitis
Pneumococcal meningitis
Adjuvant arthritis
Encephalomyelitis
Post lung transplant

It is now widely believed that it is the inflammatory response itself that is directly responsible, in part or wholly, for ARDS. There is a significant body of evidence that neutrophils are responsible for much of the clinical picture of ARDS [25-28]. Inflammation leads rapidly to sequestering of neutrophils within the pulmonary circulation and once there have the capacity to damage the host with the production of free radicals and release of enzymes in a protected local microenvironment. It is through such mechanisms that the widespread endothelial damage and resultant capillary leak typical of ARDS is believed to occur. Moreover the neutrophil can secrete the pro-inflammatory cytokines so closely linked with ARDS and neutrophil numbers in the lung correlate with the severity and outcome of ARDS. Neutrophils have been shown to be clearly pathogenic in animal models of acute lung injury [29, 30]. It is also clear however that ARDS can develop in neutropenic patients demonstrating that there is enormous redundancy in the inflammatory response and that in the presence of an excessive inflammatory response many other cells are capable of invoking such a deleterious response [31].

2.4 Anti-inflammatory responses.

Over the last few years there has been increasing focus not only on the potentially damaging effects of excessive inflammation but also on the negative regulation of the inflammatory response. The ability to switch the inflammatory process on and off is fundamental. A state of persistent activation would be life threatening while the inability to activate inflammatory cells would be equally devastating. The critical importance of activation and deactivation probably explain the huge redundancy of the system with a wide range of endogenous mediators able to promote and regulate the pro-inflammatory cascade and a similarly large number of powerful anti-inflammatory cytokines able to dampen down the inflammatory response. Naturally occurring inhibitors of TNF-α and IL-1 have been described following endotoxin administration [32, 33]. There are two soluble forms of the TNF receptors sTNFR-1 and sTNFR-II that can reduce responses to TNF-α [34]. Likewise the powerful IL-1 antagonist IL-1ra is also released in response to endotoxin and prevents cellular activation by competitive inhibition of IL-1 binding to its receptor [35]. IL-10, another cytokine associated with predominant negative regulatory properties is also released in response to LPS and other inflammatory stimuli. Along with "anti-inflammatory" cytokines other molecules that act to limit the inflammatory responses include endotoxin binding proteins and lipids. Bactericidal permeability increasing protein (BPI) and high density lipoprotein (HDL) represent two such moieties with potent LPS binding and neutralising properties that are believed to be important in limiting the inflammatory response to endotoxin [36, 37].

The balance of pro and anti-inflammatory responses is clearly of critical importance and was brilliantly highlighted by the late Roger Bone in his article entitled "Sir Isaac Newton, sepsis, SIRS, and CARS" [38]. Normal negative regulation of the inflammatory response can also be deranged and there is now good evidence that with persisting inflammation a state of immunoparesis can exist and it too is associated with a poor outcome [39].

3 Resolution of inflammation and mechanisms of repair.

The normal regulation of the inflammatory response requires not only appropriate activation and containment of the inflammatory response but also effective termination of the response when the inciting pathogen has been cleared. Neutrophils normally undergo apoptosis and are cleared by macrophages, which themselves emigrate from the inflamed site during the resolution phase [40]. Again the kinetics of macrophage clearance from the inflamed site are subject to their own regulation [41]. Thus a successful inflammatory event requires not only appropriate activation of cells and mediators with phagocytosis and removal of the inciting stimulus but also consequent elimination of the inflammatory cells and debris to allow the tissues to return to normal architecture and function.

With resolution of inflammation the tissue does not always return to normal function and in the lung interstitial and intra-alveolar fibrosis are hallmarks of the more advanced stages of acute lung injury. This may result from excessive or abnormally regulated repair mechanisms [42]. As with inflammatory mechanisms a number of different cells and mediators are involved in repair. A characteristic finding in acute lung injury is increased microvascular permeability with leak into the interstitium and airspaces of proteinacious fluid full of pro-fibrotic mediators [43]. These pro-fibrotic factors include TNF-α, TGF-β, IGF-1, PDGF, all of which are detected in the lung in pulmonary inflammatory conditions [44-48]. Another fundamental feature of ARDS is the breaching of the epithelial basement membrane with type I alveolar epithelial cell necrosis, followed by proliferation of type II cells which grow to replace the damaged surfaces [49, 50]. These epithelial cells themselves can release of powerful mitogens that can further promote fibroblast proliferation and collagen deposition. The progression to established fibrosis relies on a number of factors controlling the balance between matrix synthesis and degradation and between pro-fibrotic and inhibitory mechanisms [51, 52]. Both interferon gamma and prostaglandin E_2 can act as inhibitory cytokines to fibrotic pathways while the matrix metalloproteinases (MMP) and the tissue inhibitors of metalloproteinases (TIMPS) may also be critical in regulating the fibrotic response in ARDS [53].

References.

1.   Pajkrt D, van der Poll T, van Deventer S (1997) Inflammatory responses during human endotoxaemia. *In* Yearbook of intensive care and emergency medicine *Ed* J-L Vincent Springer. Verlag, Berlin p 14-30

2.   Bone RC, Balk RA, Cerra FB, Dellinger RP, Fein AM, Knaus WA, Schein RM, Sibbald WJ (1992) Definitions for sepsis and organ failure and guidelines for the use of innovative therapies in sepsis. The ACCP/SCCM Consensus Conference Committee. American College of Chest Physicians/Society of Critical Care Medicine. *Chest* **101**: 1644-55

3.   Bone RC (1995) Sepsis, sepsis syndrome, and the systemic inflammatory response syndrome (SIRS). Gulliver in Laputa. *JAMA* **273**: 155-6

4.   J. Bion (1999) Multiple organ failure. Pathophysiology *In* Oxford Textbook of Critical Care. *Eds.* A. Webb MJ. Shapiro M. Singer and PM. Suter. Oxford University Press. Oxford p 923-926

5.   Bone RC (1996) Immunologic dissonance: a continuing evolution in our understanding of the systemic inflammatory response syndrome (SIRS) and the multiple organ dysfunction syndrome. *Ann. Intern. Med.* **125**: 680-7

6.   Bellingan G (1999) Inflammatory cell activation in Sepsis *In* British Medical Bulletin Vol 55 (1) Intensive care medicine. *Eds.* Evans TW, Bennett D Bion JF Little RA and Young JD p12-29

7.   Bellingan G (2000) Leukocytes, friend or foe? Intensive Care Med (in press).

8.   Inflammation: basic principles and clinical correlates. (1992) Second Edition. *Eds.* Gallin JI, Goldstein IM and Snyderman R. Raven Press New York

9.   Cambrey, A.D., O.J. Kwon, A.J. Gray, N.K. Harrison, M. Yacoub, P.J. Barnes, G.J. Laurent, and K.F. Chung. (1995) Insulin-like growth factor I is a major fibroblast mitogen produced by primary cultures of human airway epithelial cells. *Clin. Sci.* **89**: 611-617.

10.   Adler, K.B., L.M. Callahan, and J.N. Evans. (1986) Cellular alterations in the alveolar wall in bleomycin-induced pulmonary fibrosis in rats. An ultrastructural morphometric study. *Am. Rev. Respir. Dis.* **133**: 1043-1048.

11.   Roberts, A.B., M.B. Sporn, R.K. Assoian, J.M. Smith, N.S. Roche, L.M. Wakefield, U.I. Heine, L.A. Liotta, V. Falanga, and J.H. Kehrl. (1986) Transforming growth factor type beta: rapid induction of fibrosis and angiogenesis in vivo and stimulation of collagen formation in vitro. *Proc. Natl. Acad. Sci. U.S.A.* **83**: 4167-4171.

12.   Condliffe AM, Kitchen E, Chilvers ER (1998) Neutrophil priming: pathophysiological consequences and underlying mechanisms. *Clin. Sci.* **94**: 461-71

13.   Ingalls RR, Heine H, Lien E, Yoshimura A, Golenbock D (1999) Lipopolysaccharide recognition, CD14, and lipopolysaccharide receptors. *Infect. Dis. Clin. North Am.* **13:** 341-53,

14.   Takeuchi O, Hoshino K, Kawai T, Sanjo H, Takada H, Ogawa T, Takeda K, Akira S Differential roles of TLR2 and TLR4 in recognition of gram-negative and gram-positive bacterial cell wall components. (1999) *Immunity* **11:** 443-9

15.   Kengatharan KM and Thiemermann C (1997) Importance of cell wall components of Gram-positive septic shock. *In* 1997 Yearbook of intensive care and emergency medicine. *Ed* J-L Vincent. Springer, Berlin p3-13

16.   Pajkrt D, van der Poll T and vandeventer SJH (1997) Inflammatory responses during human endotoxaemia *In* 1997 Yearbook of intensive care and emergency medicine. *Ed* J-L Vincent. Springer, Berlin. P14-30

17.   Suffredini AF, Reda D, Banks SM, Tropea M, Agosti JM, Miller R (1995) Effects of recombinant dimeric TNF receptor on human inflammatory responses following intravenous endotoxin administration. *J. Immunol.* **155:** 5038-45

18.   Pugin J, Ricou B, Steinberg KP, Suter PM, Martin TR. (1996) Pro-inflammatory activity in bronchoalveolar lavage fluids from patients with ARDS, a prominent role for interleukin-1. *Am. J. Respir. Crit. Care Med.* **153:** 1850-6.

19.   S.C. Donnelly *et al.* (1993) Interleukin 8 (IL-8) and the development of the adult respiratory distress syndrome (ARDS) in at-risk patient groups. *Lancet* **1341,** 643-647.

20.   Hirani N, Clay, M, Sri-pathmanathan, R, Sharkey R, Haslett, C, and Donnelly SC. (1999) A role for acute hypoxia/hyperoxia in the pathogenesis of the acute respiratory distress syndrome — an in vivo model. *Thorax* **54** S3 A13.

21.   Shanley TP, Warner RL, Ward PA (1995) The role of cytokines and adhesion molecules in the development of inflammatory injury. *Moll. Med. Today;* **1:** 40-5

22.   Huang X, Wu J, Zhu W, Pytela R, Sheppard D. (1998) Expression of the human integrin beta6 subunit in alveolar type II cells and bronchiolar epithelial cells reverses lung inflammation in beta6 knockout mice. *Am. J. Respir. Cell Moll. Biol.* **19:** 636-42.

23.   Sime PJ, Xing Z, Graham FL, Csaky KG, Gauldie J. (1997) Adenovector-mediated gene transfer of active transforming growth factor- beta1 induces prolonged severe fibrosis in rat lung. *J. Clin. Invest.;* **100:** 768-76.

24.   Tomas L. (1974) The lives of a cell. Notes of a biology watcher. New York; The Viking Press

25.   Chollet-Martin S, Jourdain B, Gibert C, Elbim C, Chastre J, Gougerot-Pocidalo MA. (1996) Interactions between neutrophils and cytokines in blood and alveolar spaces during ARDS. *Am. J. Respir. Crit. Care Med.* **154:** 594-601.

26.   Lee CT, Fein AM, Lippmann M, Holtzman H, Kimbel P, Weinbaum G. (1981) Elastolytic activity in pulmonary lavage fluid from patients with adult respiratory-distress syndrome. *N. Engl. J. Med.;* **304:** 192-6.

27.   Ward, P. A., G. 0. Till, R. Kunkel, C. Beachamp. (1983) Evidence for the role of hydroxyl radical in complement and neutrophil dependent tissue injury. *J. C/in. Invest.* **72:** 789-801.

28.   Baldwin SR, Simon RH, Grum CM, Ketai LH, Boxer LA, Devall LJ. (1986) Oxidant activity in expired breath of patients with adult respiratory distress syndrome. *Lancet.* **1(8471):**11-4

29.   Mulligan MS, Polley MJ, Bayer RJ, Nunn MF, Paulson JC, Ward PA. (1992) Neutrophil-dependent acute lung injury. Requirement for P-selectin (GMP-140). *J. Clin. Invest.* **90:** 1600-7.

30.   Rimensberger PC, Fedorko L, Cutz E, Bohn DJ. (1998) Attenuation of ventilator-induced acute lung injury in an animal model by inhibition of neutrophil adhesion by leumedins (NPC 15669). *Crit. Care Med.;* **26:** 548-55

31.   Ognibene FP, Martin SE, Parker MM, Schlesinger T, Roach P, Burch C, Shelhamer JH, Parrillo JE. (1986) Adult respiratory distress syndrome in patients with severe neutropenia. *N. Engl. J. Med.;* **315:** 547-51.

32.   Spinas GA, Bloesch D, Kaufmann MT, Keller U, Dayer JM. (1990) Induction of plasma inhibitors of interleukin 1 and TNF-alpha activity by endotoxin administration to normal humans. *Am. J. Physiol.;* **259:** R993-7.

33.   Granowitz EV, Santos AA, Poutsiaka DD, Cannon JG, Wilmore DW, Wolff SM, Dinarello CA. (1991) Production of interleukin-1-receptor antagonist during experimental endotoxaemia. *Lancet.;* **338:** 1423-4.

34.   Moldawer LL. (1993) Interleukin-1, TNF alpha and their naturally occurring antagonists in sepsis. *Blood Purif.;* **11:** 128-33.

35.   Dinarello CA, Thompson RC. (1991) Blocking IL-1: interleukin 1 receptor antagonist in vivo and in vitro. *Immunol. Today.;* **12:** 404-10.

36.   von der Mohlen MA, Kimmings AN, Wedel NI, Mevissen ML, Jansen J, Friedmann N, Lorenz TJ, Nelson BJ, White ML, Bauer R, *et al.* (1995) Inhibition of endotoxin-induced cytokine release and

neutrophil activation in humans by use of recombinant bactericidal/permeability-increasing protein. *Infect. Dis.;* **172:** 144-51.

37. Feingold KR, Funk JL, Moser AH, Shigenaga JK, Rapp JH, Grunfeld C. (1995) Role for circulating lipoproteins in protection from endotoxin toxicity. *Infect. Immun.;* **63:** 2041-6.

38. Bone RC (1996) Sir Isaac Newton, sepsis, SIRS, and CARS. *Crit. Care Med.* **24:** 1125-8

39. Docke WD, Randow F, Syrbe U, Krausch D, Asadullah K, Reinke P, Volk HD, Kox W. (1997) Monocyte deactivation in septic patients: restoration by IFN-gamma treatment. *Nat. Med.;* **3:** 678-81.

40. Haslett C. (1999) Granulocyte apoptosis and its role in the resolution and control of lung inflammation. *Am. J. Respir. Crit. Care Med.;* **160:** S5-11.

41. Bellingan GJ, Caldwell H, Howie SE, Dransfield I, Haslett C. (1996) In vivo fate of the inflammatory macrophage during the resolution of inflammation: inflammatory macrophages do not die locally, but emigrate to the draining lymph nodes. *J. Immunol.;* **157:** 2577-85.

42. Pulmonary fibrosis (1995) *Eds.* Phan SH and Thrall RS Vol 80 of Lung Biology in Health and Disease. Marcel Dekker Inc New York

43. Griffiths MJD and Evans TW (1995) Adult respiratory distress syndrome. In Respiratory Medicine (2nd Ed) Eds. Brewis RAL, Corrin, B Geddes DM and Gibson GJ. WB. Saunders Press p605-629.

44. Coker RK, Laurent GJ. (1998) Pulmonary fibrosis: cytokines in the balance. *Eur. Respir. J.* **11:** 1218-21.

45. Sime PJ, Marr RA, Gauldie D, Xing Z, Hewlett BR, Graham FL, Gauldie J. (1998) Transfer of tumor necrosis factor-alpha to rat lung induces severe pulmonary inflammation and patchy interstitial fibrogenesis with induction of transforming growth factor-beta1 and myofibroblasts. *Am. J. Pathol.;* **153:** 825-32.

46. Khalil N, Greenberg AH. (1991) The role of TGF-beta in pulmonary fibrosis. *Ciba. Found. Symp.;* **157:** 194-207;

47. Allen JT, Knight RA, Bloor CA, Spiteri MA. (1999) Enhanced insulin-like growth factor binding protein-related protein 2 (Connective tissue growth factor) expression in patients with idiopathic pulmonary fibrosis and pulmonary sarcoidosis. *Am. J. Respir. Cell Moll. Biol.;* **21:** 693-700

48. Homma S, Nagaoka I, Abe H, Takahashi K, Seyama K, Nukiwa T, Kira S. (1995) Localization of platelet-derived growth factor and insulin-like growth factor I in the fibrotic lung. *Am. J. Respir. Crit. Care Med.;* **152:** 2084-9.

49. Matsubara O, Tamura A, Ohdama S, Mark EJ. (1995) Alveolar basement membrane breaks down in diffuse alveolar damage: an immunohistochemical study. *Pathol. Int.;* **45:** 473-82.

50. Matuschak GM, Lechner AJ. (1996) Targeting the alveolar epithelium in acute lung injury: keratinocyte growth factor and regulation of the alveolar epithelial barrier. *Crit. Care Med.;* **24:** 905-7.

51. Hutchison DC. (1987) The role of proteases and antiproteases in bronchial secretions. *Eur. J. Respir. Dis. Suppl.;* **153:** 78-85.

52. Armstrong L, Thickett DR, Mansell JP, Ionescu M, Hoyle E, Clark Billinghurst R, Robin Poole A, Millar AB. (1999) Changes in Collagen Turnover in Early Acute Respiratory Distress Syndrome. *Am. J. Respir. Crit. Care Med.;* **160:** 1910-1915.

53. Ricou B, Nicod L, Lacraz S, Welgus HG, Suter PM, Dayer JM. (1996) Matrix metalloproteinases and TIMP in acute respiratory distress syndrome. *Am. J. Respir. Crit. Care Med.;* **154:** 346-52.

Acute Lung Injury: From Inflammation to Repair
G.J. Bellingan and G.J. Laurent (Eds.)
IOS Press, 2000

Nitric Oxide in Acute Inflammation

Daryl D. Rees[1] and Antonia Orsi[2]

Phytopharm Plc, Godmanchester, Cambs, UK[1] and Wolfson Institute for Biomedical Research[2], University College London, UK

1   Introduction.

In both acute and chronic inflammation physiological mechanisms, such as local and systemic vasodilatation, pyrexia and the activation of immune system limit tissue damage and remove the pathogenic insult. Although beneficial when targeted against local areas the progression to a systemic response can produce substantial haemodynamic changes, microvascular abnormalities and intracellular defects that can lead to multiple organ failure and, in severe cases such as septic shock, eventually death. These defence mechanisms are regulated by a number of diverse mediators such as bacterial products, cytokines, neuropeptides, eicosanoids and emerging evidence suggests a central role for nitric oxide (NO).

Nitric oxide is soluble in both lipid and water and diffuses freely within and between cells and, as such, can transmit signals between cells or from one part of a cell to another. It has a half-life of only a few seconds and readily reacts with oxygen free radicals [1]. In the blood, haemoglobin inactivates NO by binding it to form nitrosohaemoglobin and by catalysing the degradation of NO to nitrite and nitrate, resulting in the formation of methaemoglobin [2]. Nitric oxide forms complexes with other haem-containing proteins particularly soluble guanylyl cyclase which accounts for many of its physiological actions [3]. Nitric oxide will also bind to other plasma constituents including thiols, albumin and a variety of other proteins [4]. Thus, the fate of NO in the body will depend on its local environment.

Nitric oxide is involved in the regulation of diverse physiological processes including smooth muscle relaxation, inhibition of platelet activation, central and peripheral neurotransmission, and the cytotoxic actions of immune cells. Nitric oxide is synthesised from the guanidino nitrogen of L-Arginine, a reaction catalysed by the enzyme NO synthase. The NO synthases are a family of haem-containing enzymes of which there are three isoforms, named according to the cell type or conditions under which they were first identified - endothelial NO synthase (eNOS or type III NOS), neuronal NO synthase (nNOS or type I NOS) and an immunologically-induced NO synthase (iNOS or type II NOS). In humans, the genes encoding for these enzymes are located on chromosome 12 (eNOS) 17 (nNOS) and 7 (iNOS). Distinct genes encode for each isoform of NOS and consist of either 26 exons (iNOS and eNOS) or 29 exons (nNOS) [5,6]. Endothelial-NOS is also found in other cell types including platelets and the endocardium and nNOS is found in the brain and in "nitrergic" nerves throughout the peripheral nervous system.

The isoforms of NO synthase are large (125-155kDa), dimeric enzymes, containing both oxidative and reductive domains. The oxygenase of each subunit interacts to form the dimer and the reductase domains are attached as independent extensions. The oxygenase domain contains binding sites for L-arginine, tetrahydrobiopterin (BH4) and iron protoporphyrin IX (haem). The reductase domain binds flavin mononucleotide (FMN), flavin adenine dinucleotide (FAD), and nicotinamide adenine dinucleotide phosphate reduced form (NADPH). The reductase domain of NO synthase is similar to cytochrome P450 reductase and provides an electron shuttling transport chain from NADPH, FAD and FMN to the oxygenase domain, where oxidation of L-arginine occurs [7-9]. Molecular oxygen is also a substrate for this reaction, which proceeds via the formation of L-N^G-hydroxyarginine and results in the formation of NO with L-citrulline as the co-product.

The isoforms eNOS and nNOS are constitutive and regulated by calmodulin and require an elevation of intracellular calcium for activation. The activities of eNOS and nNOS may also be affected by phosphorylation or various post-translational modifications that regulate localisation within the cell [9,10] By contrast, iNOS is induced by inflammatory mediators and bacterial products. The iNOS isoform binds calmodulin tightly so that its activity appears functionally independent of intracellular calcium concentration. The activation of iNOS is regulated both at a transcriptional level by various factors including cytokines such as interferon γ and TNFα and at a post transcriptional level by factors such as TGF-β. The gene encoding for both human and murine iNOS contain conserved consensus sequences for nuclear factor kappa B (NF-kB), different responsive elements such as interferon responsive element (IRE) and a tumour necrosis factor responsive element (TNF-RE). Despite these similarities, there are differences in the transcriptional control of murine and human iNOS expression. In the murine system a 1.6kb region upstream of the 5' domain contains the necessary promoter sequences to induce full gene expression. However, in humans, this corresponding sequence produces little gene expression highlighting distinct differences in the requirements for iNOS induction between mouse and human.

All of the isoforms may be inhibited by naturally occurring and synthetic analogues of arginine that compete for the arginine-binding site. Endogenously found analogues include N^G-monomethyl-L-arginine (L-NMMA), [11] and N^G, N^G-dimethylarginine (asymmetric dimethylarginine; ADMA), [12] and synthetic analogues include N^G-nitro-L-arginine methyl ester (L-NAME), [13] and N-(3-(aminomethyl)benzyl) acetamidine; (1400W), [14]. The most widely studied of these, L-NMMA, is equipotent for all three isoforms and also competes with arginine for entry into the cell via the y^+ cationic amino acid transporter system [15]. Although there is close homology between the isoforms, selective inhibitors have been developed with selectivity for iNOS over eNOS conferred by substituting the guanidino function of arginine with an amidine group [14]. L-NMMA and other inhibitors of NO synthase have been used extensively as probes to characterise the physiological and pathophysiological roles of NO.

2   Physiology of nitric oxide.

2.1   Constitutive NOS and the cardiovascular system.

Nitric oxide accounts for endothelium-dependent relaxation and the release of NO from the endothelium by hormones and autocoids including acetylcholine (ACh) bradykinin, substance P and serotonin [1, 16] in arteries, arterioles, veins and venules from a wide range of species, including humans, both *in vitro* and *in vivo* [3, 17-22]. Pharmacological inhibition of NO synthase with substrate analogues such as L-NMMA not only impairs the response to 'endothelium-dependent' dilators, particularly in conduit vessels, but also causes an endothelium-dependent vasoconstriction of isolated arteries, arterioles and, to a lesser extent, veins in many species including humans [19-23]. Similarly, administration of L-NMMA *in vivo* causes widespread vasoconstriction and elevation of blood pressure [20]. In humans, infusion of L-NMMA into the brachial artery of healthy volunteers reduces resting blood flow by about 40-50% [21], and its administration intravenously increases systemic vascular resistance and blood pressure [24]. This indicates that there is a continuous generation of NO that maintains resistance vessels in a dilated state and that the cardiovascular system as a whole is in a state of active vasodilatation in both animals and humans [1,20,23].

In addition to its effects on smooth muscle within the blood vessel, NO also affects blood cells. Nitric oxide prevents the adhesion of platelets and white cells to endothelium, inhibits the aggregation of platelets and induces disaggregation of aggregated platelets [25]. Platelets themselves produce NO by the constitutive NOS, which may act as a negative feedback mechanism to inhibit platelet aggregation and adhesion [26]. The anti-aggregatory/ anti-adhesive effects of NO are mediated by activation of the soluble guanylyl cyclase and an elevation in cGMP concentrations which lead to a decrease in intracellular calcium.

2.2   Constitutive NOS and the developing lung.

In the foetus, gas exchange occurs in the placenta and not in the lung; thus, pulmonary blood flow is low. After birth, pulmonary vascular resistance falls and the pulmonary blood flow increases eight to ten fold to match systemic blood flow (300-400 ml/min/kg body weight). The decrease in pulmonary vascular resistance with oxygenation at birth is regulated by a complex and incompletely understood interplay between metabolic and mechanical factors. Vasodilatation is produced by increased shear stress or certain receptor activation including bradykinin that stimulate the generation of NO and prostacyclin (PGI_2) from the pulmonary arterial vascular endothelium [27]. Thus, NO plays an important role in the perinatal pulmonary vascular transition. Failure to undergo perinatal transition in the lungs results in persistent pulmonary hypertension of the new-born (PPHN) associated with diverse cardiopulmonary disorders, including sepsis, respiratory distress syndrome, asphyxia, congenital diaphragmatic hernias, meconium aspiration syndrome and lung. Despite the diversity of clinical diseases associated with PPHN, they share a common pathophysiology, which includes elevated pulmonary artery pressure, causing right to left shunting and severe hypoxaemia. Studies on the pathological changes in the pulmonary circulation of infant mortality associated with PPHN indicates a reduced generation of NO [28] associated endothelial cell swelling, thickened luminal membranes and an increase in muscle mass [29].

2.3   Constitutive NOS and the respiratory tract.

NO is produced by a variety of cells in the airways [30] and is detectable in animals and in tracheal gas ($\approx$ 1 ppb), oral ventilation ($\approx$ 10 ppb) and nasal ventilation ($\approx$ 20 ppb) in humans [31]. Endothelial NOS is constitutively expressed in bronchi and alveolar cells [32,33] the neuronal NOS is expressed in the trachea, bronchi and bronchioles [32,34]. Constitutive NOS is involved in the regulation of bronchial blood flow [35] and neuronally mediated bronchodilation [36-38]. In the upper respiratory tract, endogenous release of NO appears to be important in maintaining ciliary function and may provide a natural sterilizing system for the mucosa, thus reducing susceptibility to subsequent lower respiratory tract infection.

2.4   Constitutive NOS and inflammation.

As a temporary reaction to trauma or pathogenic insult, constitutive NOS is involved in the "acute phase" of inflammation, which usually spans 2-6 hours, by altering the expression of adhesion molecules on the surface of the endothelium and circulating cells [25]. Nitric oxide reduces P-selectin expression from alpha granules of platelets [39], reduces intercellular adhesion molecule -1 (ICAM-1) expression by endothelial cells [40] and ICAM-1 expression induced by IL-1 in mesangial cells [41] *in vitro*. Indeed, the basal release of NO by the vascular endothelium can decrease the adhesion of polymorpho-nuclear leukocytes (PMNs) due, at least in part, to inhibition of endothelial expression of the neutrophil ligand (CD11a/CD18), adhesion molecules including ICAM-1 and vascular cell adhesion molecule (VCAM). Consequently, rolling of leukocytes along the endothelium is inhibited and migration from the vasculature is impeded [42,43]. Endothelial NOS may also play a role in maintaining microvascular permeability and integrity. Studies have shown that inhibition of eNOS increases microvascular fluid and protein flux.

Thus the generation of NO by the constitutive NOS maintains blood vessels in a state of active vasodilatation in the systemic and pulmonary circulation, inhibits activation and adhesion of white cells and platelets and inhibits increases in vascular permeability and thus as such has a predominantly anti-inflammatory role.

3   Pathophysiology of NO.

After the initial "acute phase", inflammation progresses into a response characterised by the activation of mononuclear cells and the expression of iNOS in many cell types. Once expressed, iNOS is fully active even at low basal concentrations of calcium. Although initially described as a mechanism of macrophage cytotoxicity [11,44], important in host defence and controlling infection, it is now clear that the capacity to express iNOS in response to specific inflammatory stimuli and infection exists in virtually every cell type including macrophages, neutrophils, lymphocytes, hepatocytes, vascular endothelium, respiratory epithelium, keratinocytes, chondrocytes, fibroblasts, myocytes and astrocytes. Inducible nitric oxide synthase can be regulated both at a transcriptional level, a post- transcriptional and a post-translational level.

The combination of cytokines and microbial products required to activate iNOS and the subsequent time course of expression varies according to the type of cell, the experimental conditions and the species [45-47]. Cytokines such as TNF, IL-1, IL4 in human epithelial cells, IL2, and IFN-γ and certain microbial products induce the enzyme [45,48] whereas IL-4, IL-8, IL-10 inhibit induction [49,50]. One of the key transcriptional factors regulating iNOS expression, NF-kB, is a silent dimeric protein formed by two subunits p65 (Rel-A) and p50 (NF-kB1) and is present in the cytoplasm bound to an inhibitory protein called IkB. As a consequence of cellular activation by various immunostimulants, viruses, cytokines, reactive oxygen intermediates, and protein kinase C activators, the IkB protein undergoes phosphorylation, leading to liberation of a NF-kB heterodimer. The dimeric form enters the nucleus, where it binds to the kB site in the promoter regions of various inflammatory genes such as iNOS, inducible cyclooxygenase II (COXII), 5'-lypoxygenase, cytosolic phospholipase A2 (cPLA2), genes encoding for pro-inflammatory cytokines, adhesion molecules and receptors like α chain of IL-2 and β chain of T cell [51].

Transforming growth factor β (TGF-β) post-transcriptionally regulates iNOS expression destabilising iNOS mRNA; thus the synthesis of iNOS protein is suppressed and its degradation is accelerated [52]. TGF-β also attenuates induction of iNOS in macrophages and augments induction of iNOS by serum or tetradecanoylphorbolacetate. The stability of mRNA also appears to be reduced by IL-4, IL-8, IL-10 as well as macrophage deactivating factor.

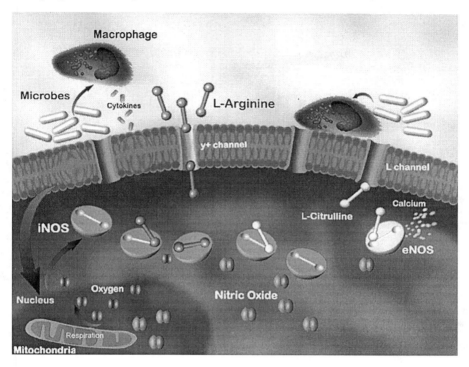

Figure 1. Microbial products and/or cytokines activate inducible NO synthase (iNOS) in a wide variety of cells. Expression of this enzyme requires *de novo* protein synthesis over several hours and large quantities of NO are produced. The iNOS isoform binds calmodulin tightly so that its activity appears functionally independent of intracellular calcium concentration. (see text for further details).

At a post-translational level, iNOS is regulated by both substrate and cofactor availability. L-arginine is the physiological nitrogen donor for NO formation so its availability represents a key controlling point. NADPH is an essential cofactor in NO synthesis, functioning as an electron donor and is upregulated by the same inflammatory mediators that induce iNOS expression. Tetrahydrobiopterin (BH$_4$) another essential cofactor in NO synthesis is involved in the binding of two inactive iNOS isomers into the active dimeric form [53].

In addition, high concentrations of NO can 'feed back' to the enzyme and inhibit its activity, providing an additional regulatory step [54].

3.1 Cellular targets.

Nitric oxide moves freely within and between cells and is also transported from the cell by putative intracellular carriers such as dinitrosyl-iron (II) complexes [55], N^G-hydroxyl-L-arginine-NO adduct [56] and glutathione-NO complex [57]. Nitric oxide then interacts at the surface or within the plasma membrane of the target cell. After diffusion into the target cell, NO can inhibit SH-dependent enzymes via S-nitrosylation such as glyceraldehyde-3-phosphate dehydrogenase [58], protein kinase C [59], phosphotyrosine protein phosphatase [60], glutathione peroxidase [61], glutathione reductase [62], methionine synthase [63] and creatine kinase [64]. Nitric oxide can inhibit certain haem-enzymes such as cytochrome P450 [65], after formation of a haem-NO adduct, a secondary oxygen-dependent reaction takes place which results in an irreversible nitration of tyrosine in the active site [66]. Nitric Oxide also mediates Fe^{2+} release from target cells, destroying Fe-S clusters in enzymes, including the citric acid cycle enzyme aconitase [67]. Other intracellular targets include proteins containing zinc-fingers such as protein kinase C [59] and alcohol dehydrogenase [68].

The mitochondria are important intracellular targets of NO. Physiological (nanomolar) concentrations of NO specifically inhibit complex IV of the respiratory chain and this inhibition is fully reversible upon removal of NO. Thus, the control of the basal respiratory rate of the cell by oxygen is modulated by nitric oxide. Pathological concentrations of exogenous NO (μM), inhibits complex IV in a reversible manner and produce a gradual and persistent inhibition of complex I [69] and other enzymes including GAPDH (our unpublished data). Peroxynitrite causes irreversible inhibition of mitochondrial respiration and damage to a variety of mitochondrial components via oxidation. Inhibition of cellular respiration by NO and ONOO- will lead to a change from aerobic to anaerobic glucose metabolism with the consequence of a reduction in ATP generation and excessive lactate formation. This inability to utilise oxygen following excessive NO production, if long lasting, could induce cell damage and lead to cell death.

Other targets of NO are at the level of the nucleus: NO can cause G/C -> A/T transition [70], mediate DNA strand breaks [71], activation of poly (ADPribose) polymerase (PARP); [72], and inhibition of DNA repair enzymes [73,74]. Nitric oxide can directly regulate inflammatory genes such as COX II [75], heat shock protein 70 (HSP70); [76], MnSOD [77] and activator protein-1 (AP-1); [78].

3.2   Endotoxin/septic shock.

Isolated blood vessels treated with cytokines and microbial products including endotoxin show a time-dependent expression of the iNOS over several hours, which begins after a lag period of approximately 2 h, depending on species. This is accompanied by an increase in the levels of cGMP in the tissue, a progressive relaxation and a hyporesponsiveness to vasoconstrictor agents over the same time course [45,79], all of which can be prevented by treatment with inhibitors of NO synthase, inhibitors of protein synthesis e.g. cycloheximide, or with glucocorticoids.

While reversal of the vascular disturbances can only be achieved with NO synthase inhibitors [45]. Thus, the increased production of NO functionally antagonises the effect of vasoconstrictor agents and plays a major role in the cytokine/microbial-induced vasoplegia. Although iNOS is expressed in both the endothelium and the smooth muscle layer, it is the latter, due to its greater mass, that is the major source of the increased NO [45,79].

In vivo studies in mice have demonstrated that administration of bacterial endotoxin stimulates the rapid release of TNFα and IL-6 which declines within 2-3 hours [80-82]. A similar cytokine profile is observed in patients with septic shock [83], and in one report following administration of endotoxin in man [84].

The administration of bacterial endotoxin in mice with the subsequent generation of several cytokines stimulates the induction of iNOS in several tissues including the heart within 4 h, that is largely over by 24 h. This is accompanied by an increase in the plasma concentrations of nitrite/nitrate over a similar time course and is closely associated with a progressive fall in blood pressure and a significantly reduced vasopressor response to noradrenaline, suggesting a similar induction profile in the heart and blood vessels [82].

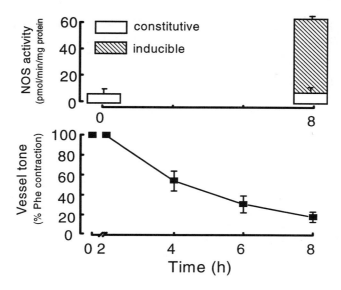

Figure 2. Endotoxin (LPS from *Salmonella typhi* 100ng/ml) activates the expression of the inducible NO synthase (NOS) and decreases the tone of the vessels precontracted with phenylephrine (phe) over a similar time course (n=10). Reproduced with permission from Rees *et al* (1990b).

Thus, in the mouse, as has been indicated for other species [85,86] including humans [87,88] the increased generation of NO from an inducible NO synthase underlies the hypotension and hyporesponsiveness to vasoconstrictor agents in endotoxin shock and may be responsible for the associated cardiac dysfunction. This is further confirmed by observations using mice lacking the inducible NO synthase in which endotoxin treatment results in a greatly reduced fall in blood pressure compared with wild type animals [82,89]. Gram-positive wall fragments including lipoteichoic acid and peptidoglycan appear to induce a similar profile [90,91].

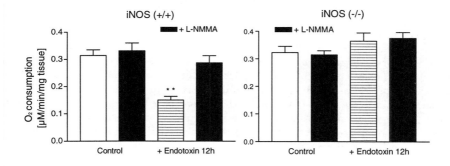

Figure 3. Endotoxin (*E. Coli*, 6 mg/kg i.v.) treatment for 12 hours *in vivo* inhibits oxygen consumption in the wild type but not in the iNOS mutant mouse. L-NMMA (300 µM) inhibited the decrease in oxygen consumption. **p< 0.01

Our studies have recently shown that in endotoxin shock, pathological inhibition of tissue oxygen consumption occurs as NO increases due to induction of iNOS. Administration of endotoxin elevates plasma nitrate concentrations, reaching a maximum at 12 h and declining thereafter in the wild type but not the iNOS mutant mice and this is associated with a decrease in oxygen consumption in the heart and liver of the wild type but not the iNOS mutant mice. In addition, L-NMMA inhibits the decrease in oxygen consumption caused by endotoxin (our unpublished data). From these an other data it is likely that the tissue dysoxia observed in patients with septic shock may be explained, at least in part, by inhibition of mitochondrial respiration due to elevated concentrations of NO.

3.3   Infection.

Bacteria including *Mycobacterium bovis* (strain *bacillus Calmette Geurin*; BCG), [92] and heat inactivated *Corynebacterium parvum* (*C. parvum*;) [47,93] induce iNOS after a period of latency of 1-2 days lasting over a period of weeks. *C. parvum* induces a sequential and differential induction of NO synthase, which is first expressed in the macrophage and the liver, followed by the spleen, heart and aorta. This suggests that following the sequestration of the bacteria by macrophages and probably Kupffer cells in the liver, their activation and subsequent generation of cytokines stimulates the induction of NO synthase in other tissues. Induction in these tissues will depend on their responses to different cytokines. In the vasculature, iNOS expression occurs 12-20 days after the administration of *C. parvum*, which coincides with the development of a small but significant hypotension. The time course of changes in plasma nitrite/nitrate, on the other hand, appears to reflect the production of NO in several different organs, predominantly the liver and macrophage in which NO synthase activity is greatest. The hypotension observed following administration of *C. parvum* is not as severe as that observed following treatment with endotoxin yet the maximum induction of NO synthase in the vessel wall appears to be greater [47,82]. One possibility is that the cardiovascular system is able to adapt and compensate for the slow onset of the expression of iNOS in the vasculature that occurs following *C. parvum* administration.

Administration of live *Pseudomonas aeruginosa* in conscious sheep leads to systemic vasodilatation without an elevation of plasma nitrate/nitrite [94]. This discrepancy may be due to the ability of live *Pseudomonas* to convert nitrite to nitrous oxide (N_2O); [95]. The ability of certain microbes to convert nitrite and nitrate to other products may also explain the lower plasma concentrations of nitrite /nitrate in human septic shock and in animal studies with live organisms compared with studies using endotoxin or heat inactivated organisms.

These studies further demonstrate that plasma concentrations of nitrite /nitrate may not always reflect iNOS activity in the vessel wall. On the other hand, administration of live *Streptococcus pyogenes* in the mouse does show an elevation of plasma nitrite /nitrate concentrations over a period of 48 hours, accompanied by a gradual fall in blood pressure, although the profile of iNOS expression in the vasculature has yet to be determined [96]. Furthermore, administration of live *Escherichia coli* for 2 hours in the conscious baboon stimulates the rapid release of TNF and IL-6 in the plasma, that declines over 24 hours with plasma endotoxin concentrations elevated over a similar time course. The plasma concentrations of nitrite/nitrate are also elevated and reach a maximum at 12 hours accompanied by a progressive fall in systemic vascular resistance (SVR). Interestingly, high concentrations of plasma nitrate at 48 hours are associated with a low SVR and death while low plasma nitrate concentrations at 48 hours are associated with a higher SVR and survival [97].

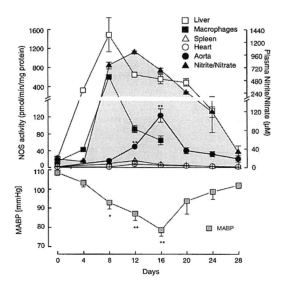

Figure 4. Time course of the sequential induction of the inducible NO synthase (iNOS). iNOS expression was measured in liver, macrophages, spleen, heart and aorta (n=3-10). Elevation of plasma concentrations of nitrite/nitrate (n=4, shaded area) and associated changes in mean arterial blood pressure (MABP; n=4-10) followed a single administration of *Corynebacterium parvum* (100 mg/kg i.p.). Day 0 represents control, untreated group. *p< 0.05, **p< 0.01. reproduced with permission from Rees (1995).

Thus these studies with microbial products or with live organisms suggest that the profile of induction of NO synthase may vary depending on the microbial strain, with a time course lasting days or weeks, which may determine the severity of the cardiovascular collapse following infection. These studies provide substantial evidence that overproduction of NO accounts for the vasodilation characteristic of septic shock [82,98] and for the hypotension induced by cytokine therapy [44]. Increased NO synthesis may also be associated with anaphylactic, and haemorrhagic shock.

Nitric oxide has been differentially implicated in the control of infection. In the early stage *Leishmania major* infection, the expression of iNOS plays different regulatory roles on the innate immune response, while in the later stage the expression of iNOS is sufficiently widespread to kill the parasites [99]. Inducible nitric oxide synthase plays a crucial role also for *Mycobacterium tuberculosis*, as demonstrated by studies with iNOS knockout (-/-) mice and iNOS inhibitors [100]. Inducible NO synthase plays different roles in murine toxoplasmosis: in the brain of iNOS mutant mice there is a great proliferation of *Toxoplasma gondii* that contributes to an early death, while the presence of iNOS in other body compartments does not control the infection [101]. Inducible NO synthase can cause immunosuppression during infection of *Mycobacterium avium:* in the iNOS mutant mouse the splenic lymphocytes have a reduced inhibition of mitogen responses in comparison with infected wild type mice [102].

3.4   White cell activation and vascular permeability.

Although inflammatory mediators and microbial products including endotoxin acutely increase microvascular permeability, the expression of iNOS in a variety of tissues following administration of endotoxin *in vivo* is associated with much greater increases in vascular leakage in those tissues. The processes by which pathological concentrations of NO produce the increase in microvascular permeability are still unclear. Nitric oxide produced from iNOS may to some extend, enhance some of the functions of the constitutive NOS, including limiting inappropriate cell adhesion. In response to microbial products, NO reduces leukocyte accumulation by affecting leukocytes directly and acts as a homeostatic regulator for leukocyte recruitment [103]. Nitric oxide may regulate the production of certain pro-inflammatory chemokines such as macrophage inflammatory protein 2, cytokine-induced neutrophil chemo-attractant (KC) and the production of IL-10 [104]. During inflammation the overproduction of NO combines also with superoxide (O_2^-) to form peroxinyitrite (ONOO$^-$), and acts as an efficient priming agent by nitration of tyrosine residues on PMN residues to alter neutrophil function [105].

Thus, the overproduction of NO may be a common mechanism by which microbial invasion, their products and cytokines lead to the excessive vasodilatation, myocardial depression, increased microvascular permeability reduced oxygen extraction and multiple organ failure observed in septic shock.

3.5   Myocardial dysfunction.

Increased NO generation consequent to induction of NO synthase may also play a role in some local inflammatory conditions of the heart, including acute myocarditis, post-myocardial infarction, dilated cardiomyopathy, heart transplant rejection [106]. Expression of iNOS is associated with myocardial depression characterised by a decrease in baseline and isoproterenol-stimulated contractility of myocardial preparations [107].

3.6   Pulmonary dysfunction.

After exposure to pro-inflammatory cytokines, the trachea, bronchi and alveolar express iNOS [32,33,108] and murine and human lung epithelial cells *in vitro* produce high concentrations of NO [109,110].

The acute respiratory distress syndrome (ARDS) represents the pulmonary manifestation of a global inflammatory process, in which widespread induction of iNOS appears to occur in the injured lung and may be an early contributor to its pathogenesis. It is characterised by a sudden, mostly generalised inflammation of the lung, which, as it proceeds, induces non-cardiogenic pulmonary oedema, pulmonary arterial hypertension, reduction of total compliance of the lung and progressive systemic hypoxaemia due to pulmonary ventilation/perfusion mismatching associated with intrapulmonary right to left shunt areas [111]. The pulmonary hypertension results from a variety of causes and may have different clinical manifestations. The causes of pulmonary hypertension include congenital heart disease with a shunt, hypoxia, recurrent pulmonary embolism, and obstruction to the pulmonary venous flow. The pulmonary hypertension causes an increase in the microvascular filtration pressure in the lung and hence development of interstitial pulmonary oedema as well as overstress and dysfunction of the right ventricle [112,113].

There is evidence that iNOS is expressed in airway epithelial cells in chronic inflammation such as asthmatic patients but not in healthy individuals [108,114,115]. This is probably due to exposure of epithelial cells to cytokines produced in asthmatic inflammation such as leukotriene D4 (LTD4). In the airways, NO [116] upregulates T-lymphocyte helper 2 cells (Th2 cells) and downregulates Th1 cells [108]. In this latter respect, NO may be considered beneficial in asthma, however, high concentrations of NO may also have deleterious effects as it may dysregulate bronchial blood flow, lead to plasma exudation in the airway [117] and stimulate the eosinophilic inflammation that is characteristic of asthma [118].

3.7   Disseminated intravascular coagulation.

Microbial products and cytokines cause the release of a wide range of cell-derived substances including procoagulants such as tissue factor. In addition cytokines induce the expression of adhesion molecules in the endothelium leading to increased thrombogenicity of these cells. These disturbances in haemostatic-thrombotic balance underlie the pathogenesis of disseminated intravascular coagulation (DIC). The increased generation of NO by the blood vessel may act as a counterbalance, attenuating the increased thrombogenicity caused by DIC and may be of particular importance in the microvasculature [25].

3.8   Nitric oxide - the link between infection and inflammation.

There appears to be an association between inflammation or infection and acute cardiovascular events [119,120]. An immediate preceding febrile respiratory infection is a major risk factor for stroke [121] and transient endotoxaemia often occurs post operatively, a time when the incidence of myocardial infarction and stroke increases [122].

The link between infection and reduction in basal or stimulated NO-mediated dilatation appears to be that of 'endothelial stunning' where inflammatory cytokines and bacterial toxins alter endothelial function for several weeks [123]. The endothelial dysfunction appears to be independent of the profound cardiovascular changes observed in septic shock and remains long after the haemodynamic alterations appear to have stabilised. Possible mechanisms involved include an effect on the stability of mRNA of eNOS, alterations of eNOS itself and other enzymes such as prostaglandins [123,124], downregulation of eNOS by large amounts of NO generated by iNOS or increased degradation of NO, such as by O_2^- [125]. Thus the endothelial damage and reduced nitric oxide activity following inflammation or infection may predispose to vasospasm, thrombosis and vessel occlusion and if prolonged possibly hypertension.

4   Pharmacology of nitric oxide.

4.1   Inhaled nitric oxide gas.

In situations in which the activity or production of NO is impaired it may be desirable to mimic or enhance the physiological generation of NO or administer NO itself. When inhaled at 5-80ppm, NO gas has been shown to reverse persistent pulmonary hypertension of the new-born [126], pulmonary hypertension induced by hypoxia [127] or after surgery, and chronic pulmonary hypertension [128,129]. The beneficial effects of NO last throughout the inhalation period and in some cases persist after termination of treatment.

In ARDS patients, inhalation of NO alleviates the pulmonary hypertension and hypoxaemia by being distributed selectively to the ventilated pulmonary areas, thus increasing blood flow preferentially to the well-ventilated alveoli and improving the ventilation-perfusion ratio. Studies in ARDS patients have shown an increase in partial arterial O_2 pressure (PaO_2) from ~150 to ~200 mmHg during inhalation of 18ppm NO.

Inhaled NO can reduce resistance in the normal lung area, diverting blood flow from regions of low oxygen tension and reducing oxygen shunt. However variable effects during NO inhalation have been observed. It appears that the major requirement is that NO should selectively reduce vascular resistance in the normally ventilated lung regions to decrease shunt flow. At the same time, it should not access poorly ventilated lung regions. The ability of NO to improve oxygenation should be enhanced when it is combined with an infused vasoconstrictor. However the combined therapy is only effective if the small pulmonary vessels are not actively constricted, but fibrotic or irreversibly narrowed as observed in the late stage of ARDS. Ideally the vasoconstrictor drug should act preferentially on vessels in poorly or unventilated lung regions, potentiating or restoring hypoxic pulmonary vasoconstriction (HPV); preserve a gradient of vascular resistance between ventilated regions receiving NO and regions where perfusion is reduced by HPV; affect only the prealveolar vessels to avoid any pulmonary venous hypertension and oedema; and have negligible effects on systemic circulation and oxygenation. Almitrine bimesylate was chosen since numerous experimental and clinical studies have shown that its action may mimic HPV. Almitrine bimesylate is a salt of a lipid-soluble molecule that is non-ionized at physiological pH. Although NO inhalation was efficient in improving PaO_2 (from ~90 mmHg to ~140 mmHg), the administration of inhaled NO and Almitrine bimesylate magnified the improvement in PaO_2 (to ~240 mmHg)[130].

In the upper respiratory tract, endogenous release of NO may provide a natural sterilizing system for the mucosa, thus reducing susceptibility to subsequent lower respiratory tract infection. This natural barrier would be lost in intubated patients and may explain their increased susceptibility to infection. It is possible that very low concentrations of inhaled NO may provide a means of limiting the susceptibility of infection in these patients.

4.2   Nitric oxide donors.

Nitric oxide donors (nitrovasodilators) have been in therapeutic use as anti-anginal agents for over 100 years. These compounds behave as prodrugs that exert their pharmacological actions after their metabolism into NO by enzymic and nonenzymic processes [131]. Cardiovascular conditions commonly treated with NO donors include stable and unstable angina, coronary vasospasm, myocardial infarction, and congestive heart failure. Scientific interest in the L-arginine: NO pathway has given rise to novel therapeutic indications for NO donors where tissue selectivity may be required. For example, S-nitrosoglutathione, in which NO is combined with a thiol group, has significant anti-platelet effects at doses that barely cause vasodilatation [132]. Selective targeting to platelets without accompanying hypotension may be of use in thrombotic disorders, where the NO donor may be used alone or in combination with other antithrombotic agents. In particular, a platelet selective NO donor may be of use in restoring the haemostatic-thrombotic balance of sepsis-induced disseminated intravascular coagulation.

4.3   Non-selective nitric oxide synthase inhibitors.

Inhibition of the synthesis of NO may be desirable in situations such as acute and chronic inflammatory/cardiovascular disorders including septic shock. Non-selective inhibitors of NO synthase such as L-NMMA restore loss of vessel tone and prevent hyporesponsiveness to vasoconstrictor agents in endotoxin-treated isolated vessels *in vitro* [45,79]. Furthermore, L-NMMA improves the haemodynamic disturbance seen in experimental models of endotoxin shock [79,82,133] but its effects on tissue damage and survival remain controversial.

Adverse responses are observed in studies where a high bolus dose of the compound is used ($\geq$ 30mg/kg) or when L-NMMA is administered at the same time as endotoxin. Indeed under these circumstances, L-NMMA precipitates glomerular thrombosis [134] and enhances vascular leak [135] in the rat. By contrast, administration of the compound several hours after endotoxin (i.e. when the inducible NO synthase is expressed) reverses the vascular leak [135]. Thus the time of administration and dose of the NO synthase inhibitor is crucial; early or complete inhibition may worsen outcome [86,136] while reduction of the overproduction of NO appears to be protective [82,86]. This dual action suggests that some NO is required to maintain homeostasis and is protective early in endotoxaemia, whereas the vast over-production that occurs later is largely damaging.

Adverse effects of L-NMMA in various animal models of septic shock may also relate to inadequate fluid resuscitation, a necessary requirement due to the vascular leak. Failure to do so leads to a hypodynamic state, with a low cardiac output and peripheral vasoconstriction that is characteristic of several studies using the dog [136]. Inhibition of NO synthase, in this situation, with the resultant further vasoconstriction would clearly be inappropriate. Indeed, after appropriate fluid resuscitation, a continuous infusion of a NO synthase inhibitor reverses the systemic vasodilatation initiated by live *Pseudomonas aeruginosa* in sheep [94] and by live *Escherichia coli* in the baboon [97]. Furthermore, in the latter model of septic shock, L-NMMA reversed the elevation of plasma concentrations of nitrite/nitrate and improved survival from 29% in the untreated group to 75% in the treated group [97].

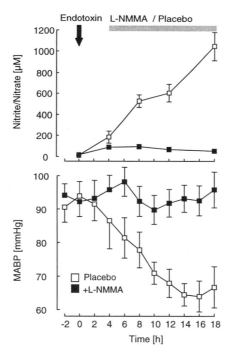

Figure 5. (a) Effect of L-NMMA (10 mg/kg/h i.v.) administered as a continuous infusion on (a) concentrations of plasma nitrite and nitrate and (b) mean arterial blood pressure (MABP) in the conscious mouse following endotoxin (E. Coli, 6 mg/kg i.v.) treatment. Reproduced with permission from Rees (1998).

In the heart, cytokines and microbial products stimulate the expression of iNOS, which contributes to the myocardial depression observed in septic shock. The reduced isoproterenol-stimulated contractility of isolated myocytes is restored by NO synthase inhibitors [137]. By contrast, in septic shock, NO synthase inhibitors, administered to reverse the low blood pressure and low systemic vascular resistance, decrease cardiac output [138,139]. The resultant reduction in heart rate and contractility, probably as a result of baroreceptor reflex action and increased afterload, reduces myocardial effectiveness. Thus, treatment of septic shock with a NO synthase inhibitor to restore blood pressure may require additional inotropic support so as to limit a potentially detrimental reduction in cardiac output.

Since NO has been implicated in microbial killing, there is the possibility that use of NO synthase inhibitors as a treatment to restore cardiovascular homeostasis in septic shock may lead to uncontrolled infection. Indeed, infection with the protozoal parasite *Leishmania major* in L-NMMA treated mice or iNOS mutant mice show greater parasite number than untreated or wild type mice [99]. By contrast, [140] have shown a decrease in *Pseudomonas* in the blood following L-NMMA treatment in a sheep model of septic shock. Further studies are required to determine the role of NO in the killing of micro-organisms in humans and whether the level of micro-organisms are altered at concentrations of NO synthase inhibitors that improve haemodynamic disturbances in septic shock.

L-NMMA has been used in clinical studies for the treatment of septic shock. Phase I and Phase II studies for L-NMMA in 32 and 312 patients respectively, demonstrates that the NO synthase inhibitor effectively restores blood pressure in patients with septic shock enabling conventional vasopressor therapy to be reduced and/or removed with inotropic support adjusted as clinically appropriate. The studies also reported that there were no apparent adverse effects on several indices of organ function [139]. Although the studies were too small to detect changes in mortality, they suggest that in a carefully controlled clinical setting, L-NMMA has the potential to be utilised as a treatment for septic shock. However, the rigid dosing schedule required may prove too inflexible for future widespread clinical use. Ongoing clinical studies are using NO synthase inhibitors to combat the hypotension following cytokine therapy in cancer patients. Whether these compounds will have therapeutic benefit in this and other low blood pressure states such as anaphylactic and haemorrhagic shock remains to be determined.

4.4. Selective iNOS inhibitors.

Selective inhibitors of iNOS are in development and may have a more useful therapeutic role by blocking excessive pathological NO generation without affecting the physiological generation of NO from eNOS and nNOS. One such compound is 7W93, which, in a conscious mouse model of endotoxin shock, has no effect on normal blood pressure but reverses endotoxin-induced decrease in blood pressure [141]. When administered as a continuous infusion either prior to or after the endotoxin-induced fall in blood pressure, 7W93 improves survival, suggesting a wider utility for the compound as a potential therapy for sepsis in addition to septic shock. Interestingly, high doses of 7W93, administered during the shock phase, increases blood pressure above normal levels suggesting that selective inhibitors of iNOS will also need to be carefully titrated. This may be due to the elevated circulating concentrations of endogenous catecholamines that follows immunological activation [142,143] and suggests that a small increase in NO production is beneficial in counterbalancing the increase in sympathetic activation. Other selective inhibitors of iNOS such as S-methyl-isothiourea have also demonstrated a survival benefit in a mouse model of shock and N-(3-(aminomethyl)benzyl) acetamidine (1400W) has shown beneficial haemodynamic effects in a rat model of endotoxin shock [144]. However, clinical uses of these compounds are limited by their severe toxicological profile unrelated to their NO synthase inhibitory properties. It seems likely that selective inhibitors of iNOS will have a greater therapeutic index and a more widespread clinical utility than non-selective inhibitors.

4.5. Glucocorticoids and anti-fungal agents.

Glucocorticoids inhibit the expression of multiple 'inflammatory' genes including the iNOS gene by suppressing transcription of mRNA through direct and indirect mechanisms. However, glucocorticoids have no effect on the activity of iNOS once expressed [45,145,146]. Most of the genes including iNOS and COX II are principally controlled by a direct interaction between glucocorticoid receptors and transcription factors that regulate their expression [147] such as NF-kB [148,149]. Glucocorticoids can also increase the transcription and expression of IkB-α, providing an additional mechanism for the control of NF-kB activation [150].

The inhibitory effect on iNOS induction occurs within the therapeutic range and may also contribute to the clinical effects of these drugs in chronic inflammatory disorders. Indeed the release of endogenous glucocorticoids during sepsis may be protective by inhibiting the expression of iNOS. Clinical data have shown that steroids are more effective if administered before or at onset of shock, therefore, these results may explain why they are more effective at preventing rather than treating the condition. Glucocorticoids also inhibit the endotoxin-induced synthesis and the release of IL-1 and TNFα and prevent the resultant hyporesponsiveness to vasoconstrictors and their associated systemic and pathological features in shock [13,47,133]. Glucocorticoids also prevent the reduction in basal or stimulated NO-mediated dilatation ('endothelial stunning') following bacterial endotoxin or cytokine administration [123].

Other clinically used drugs, which block induction, include anti-fungal imidazoles such as clotrimazole. These drugs do not block expression of the enzyme, but the expressed enzyme is non-functional following treatment [151].

5. Conclusion.

Since the discovery of NO as a biologically active molecule in 1987, it has become clear that it plays a fundamental role in the physiology and pathophysiology of inflammation. Certain clinically useful drugs are now known to act on the L-arginine: NO pathway and new uses for these agents are being explored. Novel drugs that can activate or inhibit the pathway are becoming available and will doubtless have a major impact on the future treatment of inflammatory disorders.

References.

1.   S. Moncada and E. A. Higgs, (1991) Endogenous nitric oxide: physiology, pathology and clinical relevance, *Eur. J. Clin. Invest.* **21** 361-374.
2.   A. Wennmalm, (1992) Nitric oxide (NO) in the cardiovascular system. Some physiological and evolutionary aspects, *Blood Press.* **1** 135-137.
3.   L. J. Ignarro, (1987) Contributions to a quest, *Nature* **330** 526
4.   J. S. Stamler, D. J. Singel and J. Loscalzo, (1992) Biochemistry of nitric oxide and its redox-activated forms, *Science* **258** 1898-1902.
5.   R. G. Knowles and S. Moncada, (1994) Nitric oxide synthases in mammals, *Biochem. J.* **298** 249-258.
6.   C. Nathan, (1992) Nitric oxide as a secretory product of mammalian cells, *FASEB J.* **6** 3051-3064.
7.   D. S. Bredt, C. E. Glatt, P. M. Hwang, M. Fotuhi, T. M. Dawson and S. H. Snyder, (1991) Nitric oxide synthase protein and mRNA are discretely localized in neuronal populations of the mammalian CNS together with NADPH diaphorase, *Neuron.* **7** 615-624.
8.   K. A. White and M. A. Marletta, (1992) Nitric oxide synthase is a cytochrome P-450 type hemoprotein, *Biochemistry* **31** 6627-6631.

9.   D. J. Stuehr, (1997) Structure-function aspects in the nitric oxide synthases, *Annu. Rev. Pharmacol. Toxicol.* **37** 339-359.

10.   J. B. Michel and T. Michel, (1997) The role of palmitoyl-protein thioesterase in the palmitoylation of endothelial nitric oxide synthase, *FEBS Lett.* **405** 356-362.

11.   J. B. Hibbs, Jr., Z. Vavrin and R. R. Taintor, (1987) L-arginine is required for expression of the activated macrophage effector mechanism causing selective metabolic inhibition in target cells, *J. Immunol.* **138** 550-565.

12.   R. J. MacAllister, G. S. Whitley and P. Vallance, (1994) Effects of guanidino and uremic compounds on nitric oxide pathways, *Kidney Int.* **45** 737-742.

13.   D. D. Rees, S. Cellek, R. M. Palmer and S. Moncada, (1990) Dexamethasone prevents the induction by endotoxin of a nitric oxide synthase and the associated effects on vascular tone: an insight into endotoxin shock, *Biochem. Biophys. Res. Commun.* **173** 541-547.

14.   E. P. Garvey, J. A. Oplinger, E. S. Furfine, R. J. Kiff, F. Laszlo, B. J. Whittle, R. G. Knowles and R. H. Mupanemunda, (1997) 1400W is a slow, tight binding, and highly selective inhibitor of inducible nitric-oxide synthase in vitro and in vivo Current status of inhaled nitric oxide therapy in the perinatal period, *Early Hum. Dev.* **47** 247-62

15.   R. Bogle and P. Vallance, (1995) Ketoconazole and nitric oxide, *Crit. Care Med.* **23** 600

16.   R. F. Furchgott, (1983) Role of endothelium in responses of vascular smooth muscle, *Circ. Res.* **53** 557-573.

17.   R. M. Palmer, D. S. Ashton and S. Moncada, (1988) Vascular endothelial cells synthesize nitric oxide from L-arginine, *Nature* **333** 664-666.

18.   R. F. Furchgott and P. M. Vanhoutte, (1989) Endothelium-derived relaxing and contracting factors, *FASEB J.* **3** 2007-2018.

19.   D. D. Rees, R. M. Palmer and S. Moncada, (1989) Role of endothelium-derived nitric oxide in the regulation of blood pressure, *Proc. Natl. Acad. Sci. U. S. A.* **86** 3375-3378.

20.   D. D. Rees, R. M. Palmer, H. F. Hodson and S. Moncada, (1989) A specific inhibitor of nitric oxide formation from L-arginine attenuates endothelium-dependent relaxation, *Br. J. Pharmacol.* **96** 418-424.

21.   P. Vallance, J. Collier and S. Moncada, (1989) Nitric oxide synthesised from L-arginine mediates endothelium dependent dilatation in human veins in vivo, *Cardiovasc. Res.* **23** 1053-1057.

22.   P. Vallance, J. Collier and S. Moncada, (1989) Effects of endothelium-derived nitric oxide on peripheral arteriolar tone in man, *Lancet* **2** 997-1000.

23.   A. Calver, J. Collier and P . Vallance, (1993) Nitric oxide and cardiovascular control, *Exp. Physiol.* **78** 303-326.

24.   W. G. Haynes, J. P. Noon, B. R. Walker and D. J. Webb, (1993) Inhibition of nitric oxide synthesis increases blood pressure in healthy humans, *J. Hypertens.* **11** 1375-1380.

25.   M. W. Radomski, T. Zakar and E. Salas, (1996) Nitric oxide in platelets, *Methods Enzymol.* **269: 88-107** 88-107.

26.   M. W. Radomski, R. M. Palmer and S. Moncada, Glucocorticoids inhibit the expression of an inducible, but not the constitutive, nitric oxide synthase in vascular endothelial cells, *Proc. Natl. Acad. Sci. U. S. A.* **87** (1990) 10043-10047.

27.   J. R. Fineman, S. J. Soifer and M. A. Heymann, (1995) Regulation of pulmonary vascular tone in the perinatal period, *Annu. Rev. Physiol.* **57:115-34** 115-134.

28.   J. R. Fineman and M. S. Zwass, (1995) Inhaled nitric oxide therapy for persistent pulmonary hypertension of the newborn, *Acta Paediatr. Jpn.* **37** 425-430.

29.   S. G. Haworth and L. Reid, (1976) Persistent fetal circulation: Newly recognised structural features, *J. Pediatr.* **88** 614-620.

30.   P. J. Barnes and I. Adcock, (1993) Anti-inflammatory actions of steroids: molecular mechanisms, *Trends. Pharmacol. Sci.* **14** 436-441.

31.   B. Gustafsson, L. Oland and J. S. Davison, (1997) Relationship between nitric oxide synthase activity, vasopressin and oxytocin in the brainstem and hypothalamus of the ferret, *Proc. West. Pharmacol. Soc.* **40:103-4** 103-104.

32.   L. Kobzik, D. S. Bredt, C. J. Lowenstein, J. Drazen, B. Gaston, D. Sugarbaker and J. S. Stamler, (1993) Nitric oxide synthase in human and rat lung: immunocytochemical and histochemical localization, *Am. J. Respir. Cell Moll. Biol.* **9** 371-377.

33.   K. Asano, C. B. Chee, B. Gaston, C. M. Lilly, C. Gerard, J. M. Drazen and J. S. Stamler, (1994) Constitutive and inducible nitric oxide synthase gene expression, regulation, and activity in human lung epithelial cells, *Proc. Natl. Acad. Sci. U. S. A.* **91** 10089-10093.

34.   J. K. Ward, P. J. Barnes, D. R. Springall, L. Abelli, S. Tadjkarimi, M. H. Yacoub, J. M. Polak and M. G. Belvisi, (1995) Distribution of human i-NANC bronchodilator and nitric oxide-immunoreactive nerves, *Am. J. Respir. Cell Moll. Biol.* **13** 175-184.

35. K. Alving, C. Fornhem and J. M. Lundberg, (1993) Pulmonary effects of endogenous and exogenous nitric oxide in the pig: relation to cigarette smoke inhalation, *Br. J. Pharmacol.* **110** 739-746.

36. M. G. Belvisi, C. D. Stretton, M. Miura, G. M. Verleden, S. Tadjkarimi, M. H. Yacoub and P. J. Barnes, (1992) Inhibitory NANC nerves in human tracheal smooth muscle: a quest for the neurotransmitter, *J. Appl. Physiol.* **73** 2505-2510.

37. J. M. Lundberg, A. Franco-Cereceda, Y. P. Lou, A. Modin and J. Pernow, (1994) Differential release of classical transmitters and peptides, *Adv. Second Messenger Phosphoprotein Res.* **29:223-34** 223-234.

38. B. Jain, I. Rubinstein, R. A. Robbins, K. L. Leise and J. H. Sisson, (1993) Modulation of airway epithelial cell ciliary beat frequency by nitric oxide, *Biochem. Biophys. Res. Commun.* **191** 83-88.

39. A. D. Michelson, S. E. Benoit, M. I. Furman, W. L. Breckwoldt, M. J. Rohrer, M. R. Barnard and J. Loscalzo, (1996) Effects of nitric oxide/EDRF on platelet surface glycoproteins, *Am. J. Physiol.* **270** H1640-8.

40. W. L. Biffl, E. E. Moore, F. A. Moore and C. Barnett, (1996) Nitric oxide reduces endothelial expression of intercellular adhesion molecule (ICAM)-1, *J. Surg. Res.* **63** 328-332.

41. K. Ikeda, S. Kubo, K. Hirohashi, H. Kinoshita, K. Kaneda, N. Kawada, E. F. Sato and M. Inoue, (1996) Mechanism that regulates nitric oxide production by lipopolysaccharide- stimulated rat Kupffer cells, *Physiol. Chem. Phys. Med. NMR.* **28** 239-253.

42. S. Kanwar and P. Kubes, (1995) Nitric oxide is an antiadhesive molecule for leukocytes, *New Horiz.* **3** 93-104.

43. P. Kubes, M. Suzuki and D. N. Granger, (1991) Nitric oxide: an endogenous modulator of leukocyte adhesion, *Proc. Natl. Acad. Sci. U. S. A.* **88** 4651-4655.

44. J. B. Hibbs, Jr., C. Westenfelder, R. Taintor, Z. Vavrin, C. Kablitz, R. L. Baranowski, J. H. Ward, R. L. Menlove, M. P. McMurry and J. P. Kushner, (1992) Evidence for cytokine-inducible nitric oxide synthesis from L-arginine in patients receiving interleukin-2 therapy, *J. Clin. Invest.* **89** 867-877.

45. D. D. Rees, R. M. Palmer, R. Schulz, H. F. Hodson and S. Moncada, (1990) Characterization of three inhibitors of endothelial nitric oxide synthase in vitro and in vivo, *Br. J. Pharmacol.* **101** 746-752.

46. M. Salter, R. G. Knowles and S. Moncada, (1991) Widespread tissue distribution, species distribution and changes in activity of Ca(2+)-dependent and Ca(2+)-independent nitric oxide synthases, *FEBS Lett.* **291** 145-149.

47. D. D. Rees, F. Q. Cunha, J. Assreuy, A. G. Herman and S. Moncada, (1995) Sequential induction of nitric oxide synthase by Corynebacterium parvum in different organs of the mouse, *Br. J. Pharmacol.* **114** 689-693.

48. M. W. Radomski, R. M. Palmer and S. Moncada, (1990) Characterization of the L-arginine:nitric oxide pathway in human platelets, *Br. J. Pharmacol.* **101** 325-328.

49. T. B. McCall, R. M. Palmer and S. Moncada, (1992) Interleukin-8 inhibits the induction of nitric oxide synthase in rat peritoneal neutrophils, *Biochem. Biophys. Res. Commun.* **186** 680-685.

50. V. B. Schini, W. Durante, E. Elizondo, T. Scott-Burden, D. C. Junquero, A. I. Schafer and P. M. Vanhoutte, (1992) The induction of nitric oxide synthase activity is inhibited by TGF- beta 1, PDGFAB and PDGFBB in vascular smooth muscle cells, *Eur. J. Pharmacol.* **216** 379-383.

51. P. J. Barnes and I. M. Adcock, (1997) NF-kappa B: a pivotal role in asthma and a new target for therapy, *Trends. Pharmacol. Sci.* **18** 46-50.

52. Y. Vodovotz and C. Bogdan, (1994) Control of nitric oxide synthase expression by transforming growth factor-beta: implications for homeostasis, *Prog. Growth Factor. Res.* **5** 341-351.

53. J. Wong, P. A. Vanderford, J. Winters, S. J. Soifer and J. R. Fineman, (1995) Endothelin-b receptor agonists produce pulmonary vasodilation in intact newborn lambs with pulmonary hypertension, *J. Cardiovasc. Pharmacol.* **25** 207-215.

54. J. Assreuy, F. Q. Cunha, F. Y. Liew and S. Moncada, (1993) Feedback inhibition of nitric oxide synthase activity by nitric oxide, *Br. J. Pharmacol.* **108** 833-837.

55. A. Mulsch, P. Mordvintcev, A. F. Vanin and R. Busse, (1991) The potent vasodilating and guanyl cyclase activating dinitrosyl- iron(II) complex is stored in a protein-bound form in vascular tissue and is released by thiols, *FEBS Lett.* **294** 252-256.

56. M. Hecker, C. Schott, B. Bucher, R. Busse and J. C. Stoclet, (1995) Increase in serum NG-hydroxy-L-arginine in rats treated with bacterial lipopolysaccharide, *Eur. J. Pharmacol.* **275** R1-3.

57. N. Hogg, R. J. Singh and B. Kalyanaraman, (1996)The role of glutathione in the transport and catabolism of nitric oxide, *FEBS Lett.* **382** 223-228.

58. V. Molina,L, B. McDonald, B. Reep, B. Brune, M. Di Silvio, T. R. Billiar and E. G. Lapetina, (1992 Nitric oxide-induced S-nitrosylation of glyceraldehyde-3-phosphate dehydrogenase inhibits enzymatic activity and increases endogenous ADP- ribosylation, *J. Biol. Chem.* **267** 24929-24932.

59. R. Gopalakrishna, Z. H. Chen and U. Gundimeda, (1993) Nitric oxide and nitric oxide-generating agents induce a reversible inactivation of protein kinase C activity and phorbol ester binding, *J. Biol. Chem.* **268** 27180-27185.

60.   A. Caselli, G. Camici, G. Manao, G. Moneti, L. Pazzagli, G. Cappugi and G. Ramponi, (1994) Nitric oxide causes inactivation of the low molecular weight phosphotyrosine protein phosphatase, *J. Biol. Chem.* **269** 24878-24882.

61.   M. Asahi, J. Fujii, K. Suzuki, H. G. Seo, T. Kuzuya, M. Hori, M. Tada, S. Fujii and N. Taniguchi, (1995) Inactivation of glutathione peroxidase by nitric oxide. Implication for cytotoxicity, *J. Biol. Chem.* **270** 21035-21039.

62.   A. Becker, G. Grecksch and H. Schroder, (1995) N omega-nitro-L-arginine methyl ester interferes with pentylenetetrazol- induced kindling and has no effect on changes in glutamate binding, *Brain Res.* **688** 230-232.

63.   A. Nicolaou, S. H. Kenyon, J. M. Gibbons, T. Ast and W. A. Gibbons, (1996) In vitro inactivation of mammalian methionine synthase by nitric oxide, *Eur. J. Clin. Invest.* **26** 167-170.

64.   S. S. Gross, R. G. Kilbourn and O. W. Griffith, (1996) NO in septic shock: good, bad or ugly? Learning from iNOS knockouts, *Trends. Microbiol.* **4** 47-49.

65.   J. Stadler, J. Trockfeld, W. A. Schmalix, T. Brill, J. R. Siewert, H. Greim and J. Doehmer, (1994) Inhibition of cytochromes P4501A by nitric oxide, *Proc. Natl. Acad. Sci. U. S. A.* **91** 3559-3563.

66.   L. Quaroni, J. Reglinski, R. Wolf and W. E. Smith, (1996) Interaction of nitrogen monoxide with cytochrome P-450 monitored by surface-enhanced resonance Raman scattering, *Biochim. Biophys. Acta* **1296** 5-8.

67.   J. B. Hibbs, Jr., R. R. Taintor, Z. Vavrin and E. M. Rachlin, (1988) Nitric oxide: a cytotoxic activated macrophage effector molecule, *Biochem. Biophys. Res. Commun.* **157** 87-94.

68.   D. Gergel and A. I. Cederbaum, (1996) Inhibition of the catalytic activity of alcohol dehydrogenase by nitric oxide is associated with S nitrosylation and the release of zinc, *Biochemistry* **35** 16186-94

69.   E. Clementi, (1998) Role of nitric oxide and its intracellular signalling pathways in the control of Ca2+ homeostasis, *Biochem. Pharmacol.* **55** 713-718

70.   D. A. Wink, K. S. Kasprzak, C. M. Maragos, R. K. Elespuru, M. Misra, T. M. Dunams, T. A. Cebula, W. H. Koch, A. W. Andrews and J. S. Allen, (1991) DNA deaminating ability and genotoxicity of nitric oxide and its progenitors, *Science* **254** 1001-1003.

71.   T. Nguyen, D. Brunson, C. L. Crespi, B. W. Penman, J. S. Wishnok and S. R. Tannenbaum, (1992) DNA damage and mutation in human cells exposed to nitric oxide in vitro, *Proc. Natl. Acad. Sci. U. S. A.* **89** 3030-3034.

72.   F. Zhang, J. G. White and C. Iadecola, (1994) Nitric oxide donors increase blood flow and reduce brain damage in focal ischemia: evidence that nitric oxide is beneficial in the early stages of cerebral ischemia, *J. Cereb. Blood Flow Metab.* **14** 217-226.

73.   N. S. Kwon, D. J. Stuehr and C. F. Nathan, (1991) Inhibition of tumor cell ribonucleotide reductase by macrophage-derived nitric oxide, *J. Exp. Med.* **174** 761-767.

74.   M. Lepoivre, K. Raddassi, I. Oswald, J. P. Tenu and G. Lemaire, (1991) Antiproliferative effects of NO synthase products, *Res. Immunol.* **142** 580-3; discussion 591-2.

75.   F. J. Hughes, L. D. Buttery, M. V. Hukkanen, A. O'Donnell, J. Maclouf and J. M. Polak, (!999) Cytokine-Induced prostaglandin E2 synthesis and cyclooxygenase-2 activity are regulated both by a nitric oxide-dependent and -independent mechanism in rat osteoblasts in vitro, *J. Biol. Chem.* **274** 1776-1782.

76.   I. Y. Malyshev, A. V. Malugin, E. B. Manukhina, N. P. Larionov, E. B. Malenyuk, E. V. Malysheva, V. D. Mikoyan and A. F. Vanin, (1996) Is HSP70 involved in nitric oxide-induced protection of the heart? *Physiol. Res.* **45** 267-272.

77.   Y. Lewis Molock, K. Suzuki, N. Taniguchi, D. H. Nguyen, R. J. Mason and C. W. White, (1994) Lung manganese superoxide dismutase increases during cytokine-mediated protection against pulmonary oxygen toxicity in rats, *Am. J. Respir. Cell Moll. Biol.* **10** 133-141.

78.   N. Peunova and G. Enikolopov, (1993) Amplification of calcium-induced gene transcription by nitric oxide in neuronal cells, *Nature* **364** 450-453.

79.   J. C. Stoclet, I. Fleming, G. A. Gray, G. Julou-Schaeffer, F. Schneider, C. Schott and J. R. Parratt, (1993) Nitric oxide and endotoxin, *Circulation* **(suppl. V)**, V77-V80 (Abstract)

80.   K. C. Sheehan, N. H. Ruddle and R. D. Schreiber, (1989) Generation and characterization of hamster monoclonal antibodies that neutralize murine tumor necrosis factors, *J. Immunol.* **142** 3884-3893.

81.   A. T. Silva, K. F. Bayston and J. Cohen, (1990) Prophylactic and therapeutic effects of a monoclonal antibody to tumor necrosis factor-alpha in experimental gram-negative shock, *J. Infect. Dis.* **162** 421-427.

82.   D. D. Rees, J. E. Monkhouse, D. Cambridge and S. Moncada, (1998) Nitric oxide and the haemodynamic profile of endotoxin shock in the conscious mouse, *Br. J. Pharmacol.* **124** 540-546.

83.   P. Damas, D. Ledoux, M. Nys, Y. Vrindts, D. De Groote, P. Franchimont and M. Lamy, (1992) Cytokine serum level during severe sepsis in human IL-6 as a marker of severity, *Ann. Surg.* **215** 356-362.

84. A. M. Taveira da Silva, H. C. Kaulbach, F. S. Chuidian, D. R. Lambert, A. F. Suffredini and R. L. Danner, (1993) Brief report: shock and multiple-organ dysfunction after self-administration of Salmonella endotoxin, *N. Engl. J. Med.* **328** 1457-1460.

85. C. Thiemermann and J. Vane, (1990) Inhibition of nitric oxide synthesis reduces the hypotension induced by bacterial lipopolysaccharides in the rat in vivo, *Eur. J. Pharmacol.* **182** 591-595.

86. C. E. Wright, D. D. Rees and S. Moncada, (1992)Protective and pathological roles of nitric oxide in endotoxin shock, *Cardiovasc. Res.* **26** 48-57.

87. J. B. Ochoa, A. O. Udekwu, T. R. Billiar, R. D. Curran, F. B. Cerra, R. L. Simmons and A. B. Peitzman, (1991)Nitrogen oxide levels in patients after trauma and during sepsis, *Ann. Surg.* **214** 621-626.

88. T. Evans, A. Carpenter, H. Kinderman and J. Cohen, (1993) Evidence of increased nitric oxide production in patients with the sepsis syndrome, *Circ. Shock* **41** 77-81.

89. J. D. MacMicking, C. Nathan, G. Hom, N. Chartrain, D. S. Fletcher, M. Trumbauer, K. Stevens, Q. W. Xie, K. Sokol and N. Hutchinson, (1995) Altered responses to bacterial infection and endotoxic shock in mice lacking inducible nitric oxide synthase, *Cell* **81** 641-650.

90. A. Zembowicz, S. Chlopicki, W. Radziszewski, J. R. Vane and R. J. Gryglewski, (1992) NG-hydroxy-L-arginine and hydroxyguanidine potentiate the biological activity of endothelium-derived relaxing factor released from the rabbit aorta, *Biochem. Biophys. Res. Commun.* **189** 711-716.

91. R. S. Cunha, A. M. Cabral and E. C. Vasquez, (1993) Evidence that the autonomic nervous system plays a major role in the L- NAME-induced hypertension in conscious rats, *Am. J. Hypertens.* **6** 806-809.

92. D. J. Stuehr and M. A. Marletta, (1987) Induction of nitrite/nitrate synthesis in murine macrophages by BCG infection, lymphokines, or interferon-gamma, *J. Immunol.* **139** 518-525.

93. T. R. Billiar and R. Simmons, (1992) The therapeutic use of L-arginine to increase nitric oxide production, *Nutrition.* **8** 371-373.

94. J. Meyer, L. D. Traber, S. Nelson, C. W. Lentz, H. Nakazawa, D. N. Herndon, H. Noda and D. L. Traber, (1992) Reversal of hyperdynamic response to continuous endotoxin administration by inhibition of NO synthesis, *J. Appl. Physiol.* **73** 324-328.

95. C. Braun and W. G. Zumft, (1991) Marker exchange of the structural genes for nitric oxide reductase blocks the denitrification pathway of Pseudomonas stutzeri at nitric oxide, *J. Biol. Chem.* **266** 22785-22788.

96. D. D. Rees, J. E. Monkhouse, D. Morren, N. Davies and S. Moncada, (1997) Nitric oxide induction and inhibition in the conscious mouse. *Shock* **8**, 72 (Abstract).

97. H. Redl, G. Schlag, J. Davies, D. D. Rees and R. Grover, (1997) Treatment with NO synthase inhibitor, 546C88 twelve hours after start of E. coli bacteraemia is beneficial in a baboon model of septic shock. *Shock* **8**, 52 (Abstract)

98. P. Vallance and S. Moncada, (1993) Role of endogenous nitric oxide in septic shock, *New Horiz.* **1** 77-86.

99. X. Q. Wei, I. G. Charles, A. Smith, J. Ure, G. J. Feng, F. P. Huang, D. Xu, W. Muller, S. Moncada and F. Y. Liew, (1995) Altered immune responses in mice lacking inducible nitric oxide synthase, *Nature* **375** 408-411.

100. J. MacMicking, Q. W. Xie and C. Nathan, (1997) Nitric oxide and macrophage function, *Annu. Rev. Immunol.* **15** 323-50

101. T. Scharton-Kersten, P. Caspar, A. Sher and E. Y. Denkers, (1996) Toxoplasma gondii: evidence for Interleukin-12-dependent and-independent pathways of interferon-gamma production induced by an attenuated parasite strain, *Exp. Parasitol.* **84** 102-14

102. T. M. Doherty and A. Sher, (1997) Defects in cell-mediated immunity affect chronic, but not innate, resistance of mice to Mycobacterium avium infection, *J. Immunol.* **158** 4822-4831.

103. P. Kubes, (1997) Nitric oxide and microvascular permeability: a continuing dilemma, *Eur. Respir. J.* **10** 4-5

104. M. N. Ajuebor, L. Virag, R. J. Flower, M. Perretti and C. Szabo, (1998) Role of inducible nitric oxide synthase in the regulation of neutrophil migration in zymosan-induced inflammation, *Immunology* **95** 625-630.

105. T. T. Rohn, L. K. Nelson, K. M. Sipes, S. D. Swain, K. L. Jutila and M. T. Quinn, (1999) Priming of human neutrophils by peroxynitrite: potential role in enhancement of the local inflammatory response, *J. Leukoc. Biol.* **65** 59-70.

106. A. De Belder, C. Lees, J. Martin, S. Moncada and S. Campbell, (1995) Treatment of HELLP syndrome with nitric oxide donor [letter], *Lancet* **345** 124-125.

107. J. L. Balligand, D. Ungureanu, R. A. Kelly, L. Kobzik, D. Pimental, T. Michel and T. W. Smith, (1993) Abnormal contractile function due to induction of nitric oxide synthesis in rat cardiac myocytes follows exposure to activated macrophage-conditioned medium, *J. Clin. Invest.* **91** 2314-2319.

108.   Q. Hamid, D. R. Springall, V. Riveros-Moreno, P. Chanez, P. Howarth, A. Redington, J. Bousquet, P. Godard, S. Holgate and J. M. Polak, (1993) Induction of nitric oxide synthase in asthma, *Lancet* **342** 1510-1513.

109.   R. A. Robbins, D. R. Springall, J. B. Warren, O. J. Kwon, L. D. Buttery, A. J. Wilson, I. M. Adcock, V. Riveros-Moreno, S. Moncada and J. Polak, (1994) Inducible nitric oxide synthase is increased in murine lung epithelial cells by cytokine stimulation, *Biochem. Biophys. Res. Commun.* **198** 835-843.

110.   R. A. Robbins, P. J. Barnes, D. R. Springall, J. B. Warren, O. J. Kwon, L. D. Buttery, A. J. Wilson, D. A. Geller and J. M. Polak, (1994) Expression of inducible nitric oxide in human lung epithelial cells, *Biochem. Biophys. Res. Commun.* **203** 209-218.

111.   H. Gerlach, D. Pappert, K. Lewandowski, R. Rossaint and K. J. Falke, (1993) Long-term inhalation with evaluated low doses of nitric oxide for selective improvement of oxygenation in patients with adult respiratory distress syndrome, *Intensive. Care Med.* **19** 443-449.

112.   G. J. Vlahakes, K. Turley and J. I. Hoffman, (1981) The pathophysiology of failure in acute right ventricular hypertension: haemodynamic and biochemical correlations, *Circulation* **63** 87-95.

113.   L. Gattinoni, A. Pesenti, S. Baglioni, G. Vitale, M. Rivolta and P. Pelosi, (1988) Inflammatory pulmonary oedema and positive end-expiratory pressure: correlations between imaging and physiologic studies, *J. Thorac. Imaging* **3** 59-64.

114.   V. G. Kharitonov, A. R. Sundquist and V. S. Sharma, (1994) Kinetics of nitric oxide autoxidation in aqueous solution, *J. Biol. Chem.* **269** 5881-5883.

115.   M. G. Persson, P. Agvald and L. E. Gustafsson, (1994) Detection of nitric oxide in exhaled air during administration of nitroglycerin in vivo, *Br. J. Pharmacol.* **111** 825-828.

116.   H. Kolb and V. Kolb Bachofen, (1998) Nitric oxide in autoimmune disease: cytotoxic or regulatory mediator? *Immunol. Today* **19** 556-561.

117.   H. P. Kuo, S. Liu and P. J. Barnes, (1992) The effect of endogenous nitric oxide on neurogenic plasma exudation in guinea-pig airways, *Eur. J. Pharmacol.* **221** 385-388.

118.   L. N. Heiss, J. R. Lancaster, Jr., J. A. Corbett and W. E. Goldman, (1994) Epithelial autotoxicity of nitric oxide: role in the respiratory cytopathology of pertussis, *Proc. Natl. Acad. Sci. U. S. A.* **91** 267-270.

119.   M. S. Nieminen, K. Mattila and V. Valtonen, (1993) Infection and inflammation as risk factors for myocardial infarction, *Eur. Heart J.* **14 Suppl K** 12-16.

120.   J. Syrjanen, (1993) Infection as a risk factor for cerebral infarction, *Eur. Heart J.* **14 Suppl K:17-9** 17-19.

121.   J. Syrjanen, (1988) Is there a link between infection and infarction? *Ann. Clin. Res.* **20** 151-153.

122.   R. J. Baigrie, P. M. Lamont, S. Whiting and P. J. Morris, (1993) Portal endotoxin and cytokine responses during abdominal aortic surgery, *Am. J. Surg.* **166** 248-251.

123.   K. Bhagat and P. Vallance, (1996) Inducible nitric oxide synthase in the cardiovascular system [editorial], *Heart* **75** 218-220.

124.   M. Yoshizumi, M. A. Perrella, J. C. Burnett, Jr. and M. E. Lee, (1993) Tumor necrosis factor downregulates an endothelial nitric oxide synthase mRNA by shortening its half-life, *Circ. Res.* **73** 205-209.

125.   A. Mugge, T. Peterson and D. G. Harrison, (1991) Release of nitrogen oxides from cultured bovine aortic endothelial cells is not impaired by calcium channel antagonists, *Circulation* **83** 1404-1409.

126.   S. H. Abman and J. P. Kinsella, (1995) Inhaled nitric oxide therapy of pulmonary hypertension and respiratory failure in premature and term neonates, *Adv. Pharmacol.* **34:457-74** 457-474.

127.   W. M. Zapol, (1996) Inhaled nitric oxide, *Acta Anaesthesiol. Scand. Suppl.* **109:81-3** 81-83.

128.   J. Pepke-Zaba, T. W. Higenbottam, A. T. Dinh-Xuan, D. Stone and J. Wallwork, (1991) Inhaled nitric oxide as a cause of selective pulmonary vasodilatation in pulmonary hypertension, *Lancet* **338** 1173-1174.

129.   C. G. Frostell, P. A. Lonnqvist, S. E. Sonesson, L. E. Gustafsson, G. Lohr and G. Noack, (1993) Near fatal pulmonary hypertension after surgical repair of congenital diaphragmatic hernia. Successful use of inhaled nitric oxide, *Anaesthesia* **48** 679-683.

130.   D. M. Payen, C. Gatecel and P. Plaisance, (1993) Almitrine effect on nitric oxide inhalation in adult respiratory distress syndrome, *Lancet* **341** 1664

131.   M. Feelisch, (1993) Biotransformation to nitric oxide of organic nitrates in comparison to other nitrovasodilators, *Eur. Heart J.* **14 Suppl I:123-32** 123-132.

132.   M. W. Radomski, D. D. Rees, A. Dutra and S. Moncada, (1992) S-nitroso-glutathione inhibits platelet activation in vitro and in vivo, *Br. J. Pharmacol.* **107** 745-749.

133.   C. Thiemermann, (1994) The role of the L-arginine: nitric oxide pathway in circulatory shock, *Adv. Pharmacol.* **28:45-79** 45-79.

134.   P. J. Shultz and L. Raij, (1992) Endogenously synthesized nitric oxide prevents endotoxin-induced glomerular thrombosis, *J. Clin. Invest.* **90** 1718-1725.

135.   B. J. Whittle, (1995) Nitric oxide in physiology and pathology, *Histochem. J.* **27** 727-737.

136. B. L. Cobb, K. L. Ryan, M. R. Frei, V. Guel-Gomez and G. A. Mickley, (1995) Chronic administration of L-NAME in drinking water alters working memory in rats, *Brain Res. Bull.* **38** 203-207.

137. J. L. Balligand, R. A. Kelly, P. A. Marsden, T. W. Smith and T. Michel, (1993) Control of cardiac muscle cell function by an endogenous nitric oxide signalling system, *Proc. Natl. Acad. Sci. U. S. A.* **90** 347-351.

138. R. G. Kilbourn, G. A. Fonseca, O. W. Griffith, M. Ewer, K. Price, A. Striegel, E. Jones and C. J. Logothetis, (1995) NG-methyl-L-arginine, an inhibitor of nitric oxide synthase, reverses interleukin-2-induced hypotension, *Crit. Care Med.* **23** 1018-1024.

139. R. Grover, D. Zaccardelli, G. Colice, K. Guntupalli, D. Watson and J. L. Vincent, (1995) The cardiovascular effects of 546C88 in human septic shock. *Intensive Care Med* **21**, S21 (Abstract)

140. W. Lingnau, R. McGuire, D. J. Dehring, L. D. Traber, H. A. Linares, S. H. Nelson, R. G. Kilbourn and D. L. Traber, (1996) Changes in regional hemodynamics after nitric oxide inhibition during ovine bacteraemia, *Am. J. Physiol.* **270** R207-16.

141. D. D. Rees, Inhibition of the overproduction of nitric oxide in septic shock using N^G-Methyl-L-Arginine. *In Shock, Sepsis and Organ Failure - Scavenging of nitric oxide and inhibition of its production.* pp. 1-21, Springer-Verlag, Berlin 1999.

142. C. R. Benedict and D. G. Grahame Smith, (1978) Plasma noradrenaline and adrenaline concentrations and dopamine-beta-hydroxylase activity in patients with shock due to septicaemia, trauma and haemorrhage, *Q. J. Med.* **47** 1-20.

143. S. B. Jones and F. D. Romano, (1989) Dose- and time-dependent changes in plasma catecholamines in response to endotoxin in conscious rats, *Circ. Shock* **28** 59-68.

144. G. M. Wray, C. G. Millar, C. J. Hinds and C. Thiemermann, (1998) Selective inhibition of the activity of Inducible nitric oxide synthase prevents the circulatory failure, but not the organ injury/dysfunction, caused by endotoxin, *Shock* **9** 329-335.

145. M. W. Radomski, R. M. Palmer and S. Moncada, (1990) An L-arginine/nitric oxide pathway present in human platelets regulates aggregation, *Proc. Natl. Acad. Sci. U. S. A.* **87** 5193-5197.

146. D. A. Geller and T. R. Billiar, (1993) Should surgeons clone genes? The strategy behind the cloning of the human inducible nitric oxide synthase gene, *Arch. Surg.* **128** 1212-1220.

147. P. J. Barnes, (1996) NO or no NO in asthma? *Thorax* **51** 218-220.

148. I. M. Adcock, C. R. Brown, C. M. Gelder, H. Shirasaki, M. J. Peters and P. J. Barnes, (1995) Effects of glucocorticoids on transcription factor activation in human peripheral blood mononuclear cells, *Am. J. Physiol.* **268** C331-8.

149. R. I. Scheinman, A. Gualberto, C. M. Jewell, J. A. Cidlowski and A. S. Baldwin, Jr. (1995) Characterization of mechanisms involved in transrepression of NF-kappa B by activated glucocorticoid receptors, *Moll. Cell Biol.* **15** 943-953.

150. T. Miyajima and Y. Kotake, (1995) Spin trapping agent, phenyl N-tert-butyl nitrone, inhibits induction of nitric oxide synthase in endotoxin-induced shock in mice, *Biochem. Biophys. Res. Commun.* **215** 114-121.

151. R. G. Bogle, G. S. Whitley, S. C. Soo, A. P. Johnstone and P. Vallance, (1994) Effect of anti-fungal imidazoles on mRNA levels and enzyme activity of inducible nitric oxide synthase, *Br. J. Pharmacol.* **111** 1257-1261.

Macrophage Migration Inhibitory Factor (MIF), Inflammation and Acute Lung Injury

S.C. Donnelly[1], N. Hirani[1], R. Bucala[2]

[1]*Rayne Laboratory, Respiratory Medicine Unit, University of Edinburgh, Teviot Place, Edinburgh, Scotland, UK*
[2]*The Picower Institute for Medical Research, Manhasset, New York, NY 11030, USA*

1   Introduction.

Within the inflammatory process a delicate balance exists between the potential for tissue repair and the potential for tissue injury. Macrophage migration inhibitory factor (MIF) represents a key mediator within the inflammatory response and in this chapter we will highlight recent developments in our knowledge of MIF function and activity that provides important evidence to support the rationale for an anti-MIF therapeutic strategy. The beneficial effects of inflammation, namely tissue repair, depend on a very tight control of a highly complex interplay of cellular and humoral mediators. Glucocorticoids represent one of the key endogenous modulators in controlling the inflammatory response. The repertoire of glucocorticoid effects include significant decreases in cell phagocytosis, cytotoxicity, aggregation, chemotaxis and pro-inflammatory cytokine production from specific inflammatory cell types [reviewed in 1]. These serve in general to downregulate the inflammatory response. While it is well recognised that cytokine mediators such as macrophage colony-stimulating factor (M-CSF), interferon-γ (IFN-γ) or IL-4 may attenuate specific glucocorticoid effects, until recently no mediator, induced by glucocorticoid stimulation and acting to regulate glucocorticoid action had been identified. Macrophage migration inhibitory factor (MIF) has been identified recently to fill this unique role. MIF was originally described 30 years ago as a soluble "activity" produced by activated T cells which inhibited the random migration of cultured guinea pig macrophages [2, 3]. Recently, MIF has been "re-discovered" to be a critical regulatory mediator whose secretion is induced by glucocorticoids and which has the capacity in its own right to counter regulate the inhibitory effects of glucocorticoids in the immune system [4].

2   MIF as a stress response protein.

The neuro-endocrine system, and in particular the pituitary, play a central role in the regulation of the stress response. This organ is ideally placed to integrate central and peripheral stimuli and initiate an appropriate systemic glucocorticoid response. The anterior pituitary has been identified as an important source for MIF following a systemic inflammatory response such as lipopolysaccharide (LPS) stimulation [5]. Indeed, pre-formed MIF accounts for 0.05% of total pituitary protein. By comparison, the pituitary hormones ACTH and prolactin comprise 0.2 and 0.08% respectively of total (human) pituitary protein. Immuno-electron microscopy studies of the anterior pituitary co-localize MIF to granules containing ACTH or TSH [6].

3   MIF in sepsis.

In an experimental animal model of endotoxaemia, pituitary MIF was found to significantly contribute to circulating MIF in the acute phase (< 3 hours). Indeed the content of MIF significantly decreases in specific pituitary cell types, in ACTH secreting cells by 38% and TSH producing cells by 48% [6]. When mice received an intra-peritoneal injection of LPS, not only was there a dramatic fall in the pituitary content of MIF protein but this was paralleled by a concomitant rise in plasma MIF levels and a slower, time-dependant increase in the expression of pituitary MIF mRNA [4, 5]. The addition of recombinant MIF in this mouse model of septic shock significantly potentiated lethality. Conversely, neutralizing anti-MIF antibodies was found to be fully protective to mice given a lethal LPS injection [6]. TNF–α levels were decreased by up to 35% in mice that had been protected from LPS lethality by treatment with a neutralizing anti-MIF antibody (J. Bernhagen, unpublished observations). These findings identify MIF as a key mediator in the spiral of overwhelming inflammation leading to endotoxic shock and ultimately death.

4   Cellular origins for MIF.

We have previously referred to the T-lymphocyte and anterior pituitary as being important sources for MIF. During the course of experiments on hypophysectomied, T-lymphocyte depleted mice, significant circulating MIF was detected during the early phase of endotoxaemia. This suggested that additional LPS sensitive cellular sources existed for MIF and led to the identification of the macrophage as an additional important source [7]. Like anterior pituitary cells, macrophages contain significant amounts of pre-formed MIF within intra-cellular pools (estimated by ELISA to be 2-4 fg/cell). This is in contrast to other cytokines (e.g. Il-1, TNF–α) where *de novo* mRNA generation and protein synthesis are required before significant quantities of cytokine are generated. Another difference in the regulation of MIF secretion is the concentrations of LPS required to generate MIF production. Both MIF mRNA induction and protein secretion require significantly lower concentrations of LPS (10 to 100 fold) as stimulant compared to other cytokines (e.g. TNF–α) [7].

MIF induces macrophage activation as manifested by enhanced TNF–α and nitric oxide production [7, 8]. Consequently macrophage derived MIF has the capacity to act in an autocrine fashion to promote the additional secretion of pro-inflammatory mediators which contributes to sustaining the local inflammatory reaction. Recently MIF has been described in rat renal epithelial cells from both normal and diseased states (e.g. evolving crescentic glomerulonephritis) [9]. These described additional cellular sources highlight the importance of MIF, not only within the circulation but also within tissue, in evolving inflammatory disease.

5   MIF as a counter-regulator of the glucocorticoid response.

Glucocorticoids, at low concentrations, directly induce MIF secretion from T-lymphocytes and macrophages [4]. This finding was unexpected in view of the fact that MIF acts as a pro-inflammatory cytokine and the prevailing concept that glucocorticoids inhibit the release of pro-inflammatory mediators [10–12]. Thus, MIF became the first pro-inflammatory mediator identified to be actively released from cells following glucocorticoid stimulation. Following from this, it was found that MIF acts in a dose dependant manner to override glucocorticoid inhibition of pro-inflammatory cytokine production in LPS treated monocytes [4]. Further work revealed that MIF could overcome completely the glucocorticoid protection effect in a mouse model of endotoxaemia. At higher doses of dexamethasone (> 10^{-8}M) MIF secretion is turned off and the counter regulatory effect of MIF is significantly reduced. This seems to offer the body an "escape" mechanism, allowing maximal anti-inflammatory glucocorticoid function when most required [4].

This important role of MIF in monocyte activation has been extended to T-lymphocytes and antigen-specific T-cell and B cell responses. Glucocorticoids, at low concentrations, also induce MIF secretion from T-lymphocytes. When primed T cells were incubated with antigen, MIF was found to override the glucocorticoid-mediated suppression of T cell proliferation and cytokine (IL-2, IFN-γ) production [13]. The importance of this observation was highlighted by the fact that the administration of neutralizing anti-MIF antibodies to mice at the time of immunization with a soluble antigen resulted in significant inhibition of the development of both antigen specific T cells and a primary antibody response [13].

6   MIF structure.

Human MIF is composed of 114 amino acids and has 90% amino acid sequence homology with rodent MIF. Recent work using x-ray crystallography has defined the unique structure of rat and human MIF [14, 15]. The two structures are virtually identical and may differ only in the positioning of 11 carboxyl-terminal residues. MIF protein exists as a homo trimer. Each monomer consists of two anti-parallel α-helices and six β-strands. Thus six α-helices and three β-sheets completely wrap around to form a barrel containing a solvent accessible channel.

This channel, which runs through the centre of the protein, represents a highly unusual feature of this structure. The channel diameter varies from 3-4 A at its narrowest to 15 A at each end. There is also evidence to suggest that it has a region of positive potential that may interact with negatively charged moieties. Its precise role in MIF functional activities has yet to be elucidated.

The MIF amino acid sequence shows no homology with any currently known predicted amino acid sequences. MIF does show weak primary sequence homology (27%) with the enzyme D-dopachrome tautomerase and structural homology with two recently crystallized bacterial enzymes, 4-oxalocrotonate tautomerase (4-OT) and 5-carboxymethyl-2-hydroxymuconate isomerase (CHMI) [16]. Each of these proteins catalyses an isomerization reaction, and the recent observation that MIF has enzymatic activity points to the intriguing possibility that this activity contributes to the immunological properties of MIF [17].

7   MIF in inflammatory lung disease.

MIF recently has been identified to play an important regulatory role in human disease, namely in the acute respiratory distress syndrome (ARDS) [18]. ARDS exemplifies an inflammatory disease state in which the balance within the inflammatory process has shifted quite dramatically towards excessive acute tissue injury. Inflammatory cell activation, and in particular neutrophil activation, has been implicated in early ARDS disease pathogenesis [19 - 21]. As a consequence of this overwhelming inflammatory response, disruption of the alveolar/capillary interface occurs, resulting in leakage of a protein-rich fluid into the alveolar airspaces and the clinical presentation of ARDS.

In ARDS the median circulating level of MIF was 2.45 ng/ml (range: 0 - 126.4 ng/ml). MIF was detectable via ELISA in all alveolar airspace samples, the median value was 1.19 ng/ml (range: 0.32-3.02 ng/ml). This was significantly higher than airspace samples from normal volunteers whose median value was 0.25 ng/ml (range: 0 - 0.75) (p=0.0004). Thus, significant MIF is found not only within the circulation but also close to the alveolar/capillary membrane, the loss of integrity of which is considered to be central to ARDS disease pathogenesis.

The potential of an anti-MIF therapeutic strategy was highlighted by the ability of an anti-MIF monoclonal antibody to attenuate pro-inflammatory cytokine production from ARDS alveolar cells (mean value for TNF below controls ± SD: -29% ± 6.3% and mean value for IL-8 below controls ± SD: -58% ± 23% respectively). In addition MIF was shown to override in a concentration dependant manner the inhibitory effects of steroids on activated ARDS alveolar cells. Indeed with the recognised role of MIF, both as a pro-inflammatory mediator and as a down-regulator of glucocorticoid anti-inflammatory function, these findings provide evidence for the role of MIF as a critical regulator of intra-pulmonary inflammation in ARDS disease pathogenesis.

We have recently identified eosinophils as an additional important cellular source of MIF [22]. Human unstimulated circulating eosinophils were found to contain pre-formed MIF. Stimulation of human eosinophils with phorbol myristate acetate (PMA) *in vitro* yielded significant release of MIF protein (eosinophils stimulated with PMA (100 nM; 8 h; 37 °C) released 1539 ± 435 pg/10^6 cells of MIF, unstimulated cells <142 pg/10^6cells). This stimulated release was found to be (i) concentration and time-dependent, (ii) partially blocked by the protein synthesis inhibitor cycloheximide (CXM), and (iii) significantly inhibited by the protein kinase C inhibitor Ro-31,8220. In addition, it was found that the physiological stimuli C5a and IL-5 also cause significant MIF release. Furthermore, bronchoalveolar lavage (BAL) fluid obtained from asthmatic patients contains significantly elevated levels of MIF as compared to non-atopic normal volunteers (asthmatic: 797.5 pg/ml (± 92), controls: 274 pg/ml (± 91). These results highlight the potential importance of MIF in asthma and other eosinophil-dependent inflammatory disorders.

8   Potential clinical applications.

A variable clinical response to prescribed corticosteroids is well recognised in clinical medicine. The concept of resistance to corticosteroid therapy has been documented in inflammatory disease states such as asthma [23]. In steroid resistant asthma investigators to date have largely concentrated on investigating steroid receptor characteristics specific to this group of patients [24, 25]. With the recognised ability of MIF to act not only as a pro-inflammatory mediator, but also have the unique ability to override glucocorticoid function, one could envisage a role for this mediator in blunting corticosteroid efficacy in inflammatory disease. Enhanced MIF production would result in inhibition of both endogenously-produced and exogenously-administered corticosteroid activity. This concept has important therapeutic implications. The administration of anti-MIF, with resultant removal of the MIF inhibitory influence on steroid function, could potentially form the basis of a novel strategy to combat inflammatory disease by enhancing the immunosuppressive effects of endogenously-released corticosteroids.

Indeed if one extends this concept further, an anti-MIF therapeutic strategy could have a significant steroid sparing effect. Within collected lung lavage samples from ARDS patients significant levels of MIF are found (mean: 1.19 ng/ml). It would seem reasonable to suggest that significant MIF levels would also be found in other inflammatory conditions such as asthma, inflammatory bowel disease, arthritis or contact dermatitis. Acute exacerbations of these conditions are frequently treated by steroid agents. In these situations, the combination of an anti-MIF strategy with prescribed corticosteroids could result in much lower doses of steroids being required for equivalent clinical efficacy. With the significant side effect profile of corticosteroids, any potential therapy that offers a significant steroid sparing role would be welcomed by both clinician and patient alike.

MIF was described originally as one of the first "cytokine activities" over 30 years ago. Recent advances in our knowledge of MIF structure and function highlight its exciting potential therapeutic applications in human inflammatory disease. Currently an anti-MIF therapeutic strategy would seem particularly relevant in the context both of maximising the anti-inflammatory activity of endogenous steroids and also as a steroid sparing agent. As our knowledge of MIF biology expands, particularly in relation to the regulation of MIF secretion at the transcriptional level and the characterizing of human MIF receptor(s), additional anti-MIF therapeutic "attack points" may become evident.

References.

1.   R.A. Goldstein et al. (1992) Adrenal corticosteroids. In: Gallin, JI, Goldstein IM, Snyderman R. (eds.), Inflammation: Basic Principles and Clinical Correlates (2nd edn), Raven Press, New York, pp 1061-1081.
2.   B.R. Bloom, & B. Bennett. (1966) Mechanism of a reaction in vitro associated with delayed-type hypersensitivity. Science 153, 80-82.
3.   J. David. (1966) Delayed hypersensitivity in vitro: its mediation by cell free substances formed by lymphoid cell-antigen interaction. Proc. Natl. Acad. Sci., 56, 72-77.
4.   T. Calandra et al. (1995) MIF as a glucocorticoid-induced modulator of cytokine production. Nature 377, 68-71.
5.   J. Bernhagen et al. (1993) MIF is a pituitary-derived cytokine that potentiates lethal endotoxaemia. Nature 365, 756-759.
6.   T. Nishino et al. (1995) Localization of macrophage migration inhibitory factor (MIF) to secretory granules within the corticotrophic and thyrotrophic cells of the pituitary gland. Moll Med 1, 781-788.
7.   T. Calandra et al. (1995) The macrophage is an important and previously unrecognised source of macrophage migration inhibitory factor. J. Exp. Med. 179, 1895-1902.
8.   F.Q. Cunha et al. (1993) Recombinant migration inhibitory factor induces nitric oxide synthase in murine macrophages. J Immunol 150, 1908-1912.
9   H.Y. Lan et al.. (1996) De novo renal expression of macrophage migration inhibitory factor during the development of rat crescenteric glomerulonephritis. Am J Path 149, 1119-1127.
10.   B. Beutler et al. (1986) Control of cachectin (tumor necrosis factor) synthesis: mechanisms of endotoxin resistance. Science 270, 977-980.
11.   R.I. Scheinman et al. (1995) Role of transcriptional activation of IκBα in mediation of immunosuppression of glucocorticoids. Science 270, 283-290.
12.   N. Auphan et al. (1995) Immunosuppression by glucocorticoids: inhibition of NF-kb activity through induction of IkB synthesis. Science 270, 286-290.
13.   M. Bacher et al. (1996) An essential regulatory role for MIF in T-cell activation. Proc. Natl. Acad. Sci. 93, 7849-7854.
14.   H.W. Sun et al. (1996) Crystal structure at 2.6-A resolution of human macrophage migration inhibitory factor. Proc. Natl. Acad. Sci. 93, 5191-5196.

15.   M. Suzuki *et al.* (1996) Crystal structure of the macrophage migration inhibitory factor from rat liver. *Nature Struct. Biol.* **3**, 259-266,

16.   H.S. Subramanya *et al.* (1996) Enzymatic ketonization of 2-hydroxymuconate: specificity and mechanism investigated by the crystal structures of two isomerases. *Biochemistry* **35**, 792-802.

17.   E. Rosengren *et al.* (1996)The immunoregulatory mediator macrophage migration inhibitory factor (MIF) catalyzes a tautomerization reaction. *Moll Med* **2**, 143-149.

18.   S.C. Donnelly *et al.* (1997) Regulatory role for macrophage migration inhibitory factor in acute respiratory distress syndrome. *Nature Med* **3**, 320-323.

19.   S. C Donnelly *et al.* (1994) Role of selectins in development of adult respiratory distress syndrome. *Lancet* **344**, 215-219.

20.   S.C. Donnelly *et al.* (1993) Interleukin 8 (IL-8) and the development of the adult respiratory distress syndrome (ARDS) in at-risk patient groups. *Lancet* **1341**, 643-647.

21.   S. C. Donnelly and C. Haslett. (1992) Cellular mechanisms of acute lung injury: implications for future treatment in the adult respiratory distress syndrome. *Thorax* **47**, 260-263.

22.   A.G Rossi *et al.* (1998) Eosinophils are a source for macrophage migration inhibitory factor (MIF) - potential role in asthma. J Clin Invest **101**, 2869-2874.

23.   P.J. Barnes *et al.* (1992) Glucocorticoid resistance in asthma. *Am J Respir & Crit Care Med* **152**, S125-S142.

24.   I.M. Adcock *et al.* (1995) Abnormal glucocorticoid receptor-activator protein - 1 interaction in steroid resistant asthma. *J. Exp. Med.* **182**, 1951-1958.

25.   I.M Adcock and P.J. Barnes. (1995) Steroid resistant asthma. *Q J M* **88**, 455-568.

Acute Lung Injury: From Inflammation to Repair
G.J. Bellingan and G.J. Laurent (Eds.)
IOS Press, 2000

Oxidative Stress in COPD

William MacNee

Medical & Radiological Sciences, ELEGI, Colt Research Laboratories,
Wilkie Building, University of Edinburgh, Edinburgh, Scotland, UK

Abstract: Oxidative stress results from an oxidant/antioxidant imbalance, in favour of oxidants. There is substantial evidence that oxidative stress plays an important role in the pathogenesis of chronic obstructive pulmonary disease (COPD). A large number of studies have shown an increased oxidant burden and consequently increased markers of oxidative stress in the airspaces, breath, blood and urine in smokers and patients with COPD. Several consequences of oxidative stress are important in the pathogenesis of COPD. These include oxidative inactivation of antiproteinases, airspace epithelial injury, increased sequestration of neutrophils in the pulmonary microvasculature, and gene expression of pro-inflammatory mediators, through the activation of redox sensitive transcriptions factors, such as NF-κB and AP-1, which regulate the genes for pro-inflammatory mediators and protective antioxidant gene expression.

Oxidative stress can result from oxidants present in cigarette smoke, or from the release of increased amounts of reactive oxygen species from leukocytes, both in the airspaces and in the blood. Depletion or deficiency in antioxidants may contribute to oxidative stress. Dietary deficiency in antioxidants is related to the development of airflow limitation and hence dietary supplementation may be a beneficial therapeutic intervention in this condition. The use of antioxidants with good bioavailability or molecules which have antioxidant enzyme activity may be treatments which not only protect against the direct injurious effects of oxidants, but may fundamentally alter the inflammatory events which are thought to play an important part in the pathogenesis of COPD.

Key words: Chronic obstructive pulmonary disease, oxidants, antioxidant, and reactive oxidant species.

1   Introduction.

Chronic Obstructive Pulmonary Disease (COPD) produces considerable morbidity and mortality world-wide [1]. It is a slowly progressive condition characterised by airflow limitation, which is largely irreversible [2]. A smoking history of at least 20 pack years is usual, reflecting the fact that smoking is the main aetiological factor in this condition, far outweighing any of the other risk factors. The pathogenesis of COPD is therefore strongly linked to the effects of cigarette smoke on the lungs. Cigarette smoke contains 10^{17} molecules per puff [3]. The proposal that an oxidant/antioxidant imbalance occurs in smokers and in patients with COPD, as part of the pathogenesis of this condition, as received increasing research attention in recent years [4].

2   Proteinase/antiproteinase hypothesis of the pathogenesis of emphysema.

The concept that a proteinase/ antiproteinase imbalance is the critical mechanism in the pathogenesis of emphysema in smokers developed from studies which showed the early

development of emphysema in α_1-Anti-trypsin (α_1 AT) deficient subjects. In the case of smokers with normal levels of α_1-AT several mechanisms may be involved:
The elastase burden may be increased, as a result of increased recruitment of leukocytes to the lungs.
There may be a functional deficiency of α_1-AT, due to inactivation of α_1-AT in the lungs or failure to mount an adequate increased level during lung inflammation.
A deficiency of other antiproteases and/or an increase in other proteases may contribute to the protease/antiprotease imbalance in the lungs.
The repair mechanisms for proteolytic damage may be inadequate or inactivated.

A large body of literature has amassed in an attempt to prove the protease /antiprotease theory of the pathogenesis of emphysema. It is clear from the hypothesis that the view of an imbalance between an increased elastase burden in the lungs and a functional 'deficiency' of α_1-AT due to its inactivation by oxidants, is an over simplification, not least, as described above, because other proteinases and other antiproteinases are likely to have a role. However, the key events in the pathogenic processes that have been investigated in humans are:
a. Increased elastase burden in the lungs due to increased recruitment of leukocytes
b. Decreased functional antiproteinases in the airspace lining fluid.

2.1   Increased elastase burden.

It has been proposed that variations in the elastase content of neutrophils contributes to the increased elastase burden in the lungs of smokers. Early studies suggested that neutrophil elastase content was increased in patients with COPD [5] but not, interestingly, in patients with alpha-1-antitrypsin deficiency [6]. Although subsequent studies have shown that neutrophils from subjects with COPD demonstrate increased extracellular proteolytic activity, they have not confirmed that the elastase content of the neutrophils is increased [7]. However, other studies have suggested that variations in elastase content may help to explain why not all patients with PIZ alpha-1-antitrypsin deficiency develop emphysema [8]. Thus the hypothesis that variations in elastase content are important in the pathogenesis of emphysema remains unproven.

Another way in which the elastase burden could be enhanced in cigarette smokers is if neutrophils from smokers demonstrated enhanced degranulation and therefore release of elastase. There is some evidence to support this, since neutrophils isolated from patients with emphysema show greater elastase-induced fibronectin degradation *in vitro* than cells from control subjects matched for age and smoking history [7,9].

2.2   Inactivation of antiproteinases.

Central to the development of a protease-antiprotease imbalance in smokers is the inactivation of antiproteinases by oxidants in cigarette smoke or released by leukocytes. Early studies showed that the function of α_1-1-antitrypsin in bronchoalveolar lavage was reduced by around 40% in smokers, compared with non-smokers [10]. This "functional α_1-1-AT deficiency" is thought to be due to inactivation of the α_1-1-AT by oxidation of the methionine residue at its active site [11,12] by oxidants in cigarette smoke. Another major inhibitor of neutrophil elastase (NE) is secretory leukoprotease inhibitor (SLPI), which can also be inactivated by oxidants [13,14].

This theory was supported by *in vitro* studies showing loss of α_1-1-AT inhibitory capacity when treated with oxidants [15], including cigarette smoke [16]. In addition oxidation of the methionine residue in α_1-1-AT was confirmed in the lungs of healthy smokers [17]. These studies supported the concept of inactivation of α_1-1-AT by oxidation of the active site of the protein. Other studies showed that macrophages from the lungs of smokers release increased amounts of reactive oxygen species, which could also inactivate α_1-1-AT *in vitro* [12,18]. However, most of the α_1-1-AT in the lung lining fluid in cigarette smokers remains active and is therefore still capable of protecting the lungs against the increased protease burden. Later studies have provided conflicting data on whether α_1-1-AT function in bronchoalveolar lavage is altered in cigarette smokers [19]. This may be due to technical differences between the studies which may have affected α_1-1-AT function. In addition the observation that oxidation of α_1-1-AT occurs in bronchoalveolar lavage in smokers has not been confirmed [20].

Studies which have assessed the acute effects of cigarette smoking on the functional activity of α_1-1-AT in bronchoalveolar lavage fluid, and have shown a transient, but non-significant fall in the anti-protease activity of bronchoalveolar lavage fluid one hour after smoking [21]. Thus studies assessing the function of α_1-1-AT in either chronic or acute cigarette smoking have failed to produce a clear picture. A further hypothesis has been developed to explain this conflicting data, and has invoked a contributory role for other antiproteases, such as antileukoprotease, or by observing more subtle changes, for example a decrease in the association rate constant of α_1-1-AT for neutrophil elastase which may contribute to elastin degradation [22].

Oxidative stress may have injurious effects on several target cells in smokers and in patients with COPD. Recent data also indicates that oxidative stress acts as a trigger for the up-regulation of pro-inflammatory genes and protective mechanisms such as the upregulation of genes for antioxidants (see below).

3   Increased oxidant burden in smokers and patients with COPD.

3.1   Oxidants in cigarette smoke.

Amongst the complex mixture of over 4,700 chemical compounds in cigarette smoke are high concentrations of free radicals and other oxidants [3,23]. Free radicals are present in both the tar and the gas phases of cigarette smoke. The gas-phase of cigarette smoke contains approximately 10^{15} radicals per puff, primarily of the alkyl and peroxyl types. Nitric oxide is another oxidant which is present in cigarette smoke in concentrations of 500-1000 ppm [24]. Nitric oxide (NO·) reacts quickly with the superoxide anion (O_2^-) to form peroxynitrite (ONOO), and with peroxyl radicals to give alkyl peroxynitrites (ROONO).

The tar phase of cigarette contains radicals which are more stable and are predominantly organic, such as the semiquinone radical, which can react with oxygen to produce O_2^-. The tar phase also contains the hydroxyl radical (OH) and hydrogen peroxide (H_2O_2) [24]. It is also an effective metal chelator and can bind iron to produce the tar-semiquinone + tar-Fe^{2+}, which can generate H_2O_2 [25].

The epithelial lining fluid (ELF) in the lungs may be effective in immediately quenching the short-lived radicals in the gas phase of cigarette smoke. However, redox reactions in cigarette smoke condensate, which forms in the epithelial lining fluid, may continue to produce reactive oxygen species (ROS) for a considerable time.

3.2   Cell-derived oxidants.

The increased oxidative burden produced by inhaling cigarette smoke can be further enhanced in the lungs of cigarette smokers by the release of oxygen radicals from the influx and activation of inflammatory leukocytes, both neutrophils and macrophages, which is known to occur in the lungs of cigarette smokers [26]. Increased amounts of oxidants such as O_2^- and H_2O_2 have been shown to be released from smokers, compared with non-smokers leukocytes [27].

Iron is a critical element in many oxidative reactions. The generation of oxidants in epithelial lining fluid in smokers is further enhanced by the presence of increased amounts of free iron in the airspaces [28]. The intracellular iron content of alveolar macrophages is increased in cigarette smokers and is increased further in those who develop chronic bronchitis, compared with non-smokers [29]. Furthermore, macrophages from smokers release more free iron *in vitro* than those from non-smokers [30].

Free iron in the ferrous form can take part in the Fenton and Haber-Weiss reactions, which generate the hydroxyl radical, a free radical which is extremely damaging to all tissues, particularly to cell membranes, producing lipid peroxidation.

3.3   Oxidant damage.

Direct oxidative damage to components of the lung matrix (such as elastin and collagen) can results from oxidants in cigarette smoke. Elastin synthesis and repair can also be impaired by cigarette smoke [31], which can augment proteolytic damage to matrix components and thus enhance the development of emphysema.

3.4   Oxidative stress in the alveolar space.

All tissues are vulnerable to oxidant damage but, by virtue of its direct contact with the environment, the airspace epithelial surface of the lung is particularly vulnerable. The respiratory tract lining fluids (RTLF) forms an interface between the epithelial cells and the external environment and thus constitutes a "first line of defence" against inhaled oxidants. Injury to the respiratory tract epithelial cells from cigarette smoke could occur by at least 3 processes: a) a direct toxic interaction of airspace cells with constituents of cigarette smoke (including free radicals) which have penetrated the protective antioxidant shield of the RTLF; b) damage to the cells by toxic reactive products generated by interaction between cigarette smoke and RTLFs; and c) reactions occurring subsequent to activation of inflammatory-immune processes initiated by a) and/or b) [32-34].

Injury to the epithelium may be an important early event following exposure to cigarette smoke, manifest as an increase in airspace epithelial permeability [35]. Lannan and colleagues [36] demonstrated the injurious effect of both whole and vapour phases of cigarette smoke on human alveolar epithelial cell monolayers, as shown by increased epithelial cell detachment, decreased cell adherence and increased cell lysis. These effects were in part oxidant-mediated since the antioxidant glutathione (GSH) conferred protection against these injurious effects of cigarette smoke in concentrations (500µM) present in the epithelial lining fluid.

Extra- and intra-cellular glutathione appears to be critical to the maintenance of epithelial integrity following exposure to cigarette smoke. This was shown in studies by Li et al [37, 38] and Rahman et al [39] which demonstrate that the increased epithelial permeability of epithelial cell monolayers *in vitro*, and in rat lungs *in vivo* following exposure to cigarette smoke condensate, was associated with profound changes in the homeostasis of the antioxidant glutathione. Intracellular and total lung glutathione levels were considerably decreased, concomitant with a decrease in the activities of the enzymes involved in the GSH redox cycle such as glutathione peroxidase and glucose-6-phosphate dehydrogenase following exposure to cigarette smoke condensate. Depletion of lung GSH alone, by treatment with the glutathione synthesis inhibitor buthionine sulphoxamine, can induce increased airspace epithelial permeability both *in vitro* and *in vivo* [38-40].

These *in vitro* and animal studies are paralleled by human studies demonstrating increased epithelial permeability in chronic smokers compared with non-smokers, as measured by increased [99m]technetium-diethylenetriaminepentacetate, ([99m] Tc-DTPA) lung clearance, with a further increase in [99m] Tc-DTPA clearance following acute smoking [27] (Figure 1). Thus cigarette smoke has a detrimental effect on the alveolar epithelial cell function which is, in part, oxidant-mediated, since antioxidants provide protection against this injurious event.

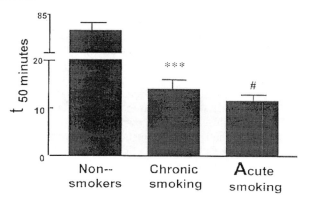

Figure 1. Mean (Bars SD) values for ^{99m}Tc-DTPA lung clearance (time to 50% clearance - t_{50}) in non-smokers, chronic smokers and the acute effects of smoking (*** p<0.05)

The oxidant burden in lungs may be further enhanced in smokers by the increased numbers of neutrophils (by 10-fold) and macrophages (by 2-4 fold) [41,42] in the alveolar space. *In vitro* studies have shown that alveolar leukocytes from cigarette smokers spontaneously release increased amounts of oxidants, such as O_2^- and H_2O_2 ,compared to those from non-smokers [43-49]. Recent evidence from bronchial biopsy and lung resection studies indicates that increased numbers of neutrophils are present in both bronchial and alveolar walls in smokers with moderately severe COPD [50].

Much research has focussed on the presence and function of airspace leukocytes in chronic smokers, studied by bronchoalveolar lavage. However, the dynamics of the events, which occur repeatedly during the act of smoking, may be critical to the pathogenesis of smoking-induced lung injury. In the breath levels of the oxidants hydrogen peroxide and nitric oxide have been shown to be increased in patients with both stable and acute COPD, in the case of hydrogen peroxide [51] and in exacerbations of the condition, the case of nitric oxide [52].

Alveolar leukocytes from smokers and patients with chronic bronchitis have increased ability to release oxygen radicals, compared with those from healthy controls [53] activity of Xanthine/Xanthine oxidase, which generates superoxide anion has also been shown to be increased in the bronchoalveolar lavage fluid from patients with COPD [54].

3.5 Oxidative stress in the circulation.

The first step in the recruitment of neutrophils in to the airspaces is the sequestration of these cells in the lung microcirculation [55]. Under normal circumstances, this occurs in the pulmonary capillary bed, as a result of the size differential between neutrophils (average diameter 7 μM) and pulmonary capillary segments (average diameter 5 μM). Thus a proportion of the circulating neutrophils have to deform in order to negotiate the smaller capillary segments. There are approximately 3×10^8 alveoli with approximately 3×10^{11} capillary segments in their walls, i.e. 1000 capillary segments per alveolus. It has been estimated that the average pathway for a neutrophil from the arteriole to the venule comprises six of these short interconnected pulmonary capillary segments [56]. Studies using a variety of techniques, including radio-labelled or fluorescently labelled neutrophils, have supported the idea that the lungs contain a large pool of non-circulating neutrophils, which are either retained or slowly moving within the pulmonary microcirculation. These studies, using cells harvested from the blood, labelled *in vitro* and re-injected, are supported by morphometric techniques, which indicate that native, unlabelled neutrophils are present in the pulmonary capillaries in greater numbers than would be expected for the numbers of erythrocytes [55,56]. In healthy subjects, radio-labelled neutrophil studies indicate that a proportion of neutrophils are normally delayed in the pulmonary circulation, compared to radio-labelled erythrocytes [55]. Autoradiographs of lung sections following re-injection or morphometric techniques to count radio-labelled cells on histological section of the lungs, have shown that the delay or sequestration of neutrophils occurs in the pulmonary capillary bed [55]. Studies in normal subjects have shown a correlation between neutrophil deformability measured *in vitro* and the subsequent sequestration of these cells in the pulmonary microcirculation following their re-injection — the less deformable the cells the greater the sequestration of these cells in the pulmonary microcirculation [57]. Thus a degree of neutrophil sequestration occurs in normal lungs, because of the necessity of these cells to deform in order to pass through the pulmonary capillary segments. This provides a mechanism for the creation of a pool of sequestered or non-circulating cells in the pulmonary microcirculation, without the need to invoke margination of neutrophils in the post capillary venules, which creates a non-circulating pool of cells in the systemic circulation [55,56]. The sequestration of neutrophils in the pulmonary capillaries allows time for the neutrophils to interact with the pulmonary capillary endothelium, resulting in their firm adherence to the endothelium. This event is mediated by the upregulation of adhesion molecules on the surfaces of both the neutrophils and endothelial cells, as a prelude to transmigration across the alveolar capillary membrane into the interstitium and airspaces of the lungs in response to inflammation or infection. Any circumstances which lead to a decrease in neutrophil deformability will potentially increase neutrophil sequestration in the lungs. This may be initiated by an inappropriate inflammatory response and may result in neutrophil-induced lung injury.

Decreased neutrophil deformability occurs in cell activation, due to the assembly of the cytoskeleton, in particular the polymerisation of microfilaments (F actin), resulting in cell stiffening. Neutrophils can be activated while in transit in the pulmonary microcirculation by a number of mediators, including cytokines released from resident lung cells, alveolar macrophages, epithelial and endothelial cells. Noxious inhaled agents, such as cigarette smoke and other air pollutants, could influence the transit of cells in the pulmonary capillary bed. Studies in man using radio-labelled neutrophils and red cells show a transient increase in neutrophil sequestration in the lungs during smoking [58], which returns to normal after cessation of smoking. Using an *in vitro* positive pressure cell filtration technique it has been shown that cells exposed to cigarette smoke *in vitro* decrease their deformability [59]. A similar decrease in deformability can be demonstrated *in vivo* for neutrophils in blood obtained from subjects who are actively smoking (Figure 2) [60]. Since each puff of cigarette smoke contains 10^{16} oxidant molecules, it has been suggested that the effect of cigarette smoke on neutrophil deformability is oxidant-mediated. Support for this hypothesis comes from *in vitro* studies, which show that the decrease neutrophil deformability induced by cigarette smoke exposure is abolished by antioxidants, such as glutathione [59]. There is evidence of oxidative stress reaching the circulation during cigarette smoking which could decrease the deformability of neutrophils, so increasing their sequestration in the pulmonary microcirculation [60]. Oxidants appear to affect neutrophil deformability by altering the cytoskeleton by polymerising actin [59]. Thus cigarette smoking increases neutrophil sequestration in the pulmonary microcirculation, at least in part, by decreasing neutrophil deformability.

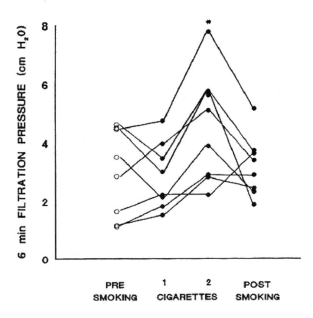

Figure 2. Effect of cigarette smoking on *in vitro* 6 minute filtration pressure of neutrophils harvested from arterial blood as a measure of cell deformability, in 8 healthy cigarette smokers. Following 2 cigarettes the filtration pressure increased and hence neutrophil deformability decreased (*p<0.05 compared with control).

Once sequestered, components of cigarette smoke can alter neutrophil adhesion to endothelium by upregulating CD18 integrins [61,62]. Cigarette smoke has also been shown to alter neutrophil adhesion [61,62]. Inhalation of cigarette smoke by hamsters increases neutrophil adhesion to the endothelium of both arterioles and venules [61]. This increased neutrophil adhesion is thought to be mediated by superoxide anion derived from cigarette smoke, since it was inhibited by pre-treatment with CuZnSOD [61]. Neutrophils sequestered in the pulmonary circulation of the rabbit following cigarette smoke inhalation also show increased expression of CD18 integrins [62], which is known to upregulate the NADPH oxidase-O_2^- generating system [63].

Increased expression of adhesion molecules in smoke exposed animals may result from the secondary inflammatory effects of smoking, through the release of cytokines, since direct smoke exposure *in vitro* does not produce increased expression of neutrophil adhesion molecules, nor does it enhanced functional adherence [64]. Thus several mechanisms involving oxidants cause neutrophil sequestration in the pulmonary microcirculation in smokers. Oxidant-mediated mechanisms may also result in the increased sequestration of neutrophils, which occurs in the microcirculation during exacerbations of COPD [57] and this may also be oxidant-induced [65].

These sequestered neutrophils may subsequently respond to the chemotactic components in cigarette smoke and become more adhesive to pulmonary vascular endothelial cells, in preparation for migration into the airspaces. Studies in animal models of smoke exposure have shown increased neutrophil sequestration in the pulmonary microcirculation in situ, associated with upregulation of adhesion molecules on the surface of these cells [62]. Activation of neutrophils sequestered in the pulmonary microvasculature could also induce the release of reactive oxygen intermediates and proteases within the micro-environment with limited access for free radical scavengers and antiproteases. Thus destruction of the alveolar wall, as occurs in emphysema, could result from a proteolytic insult derived from the intra-vascular space, without the need for the neutrophils to migrate into the airspaces.

As indicated above, several studies have shown that there are increased numbers of neutrophils in the bronchoalveolar lavage in chronic cigarette smokers [4]. Neutrophil sequestration in the microcirculation, allows chemotaxis to occur. Nicotine itself is chemotactic [66]. Smoke exposure in animals [67] and in humans results in increased chemotactic activity or levels of chemotactic factors in the airspaces [68].

Ex vivo studies however have suggested that epithelial cells from cigarette smokers and patients with COPD are less likely to release chemotactic factors in response to stimuli compared to non-smokers [69]. Alveolar macrophages can also release chemotactic factors. For example, alveolar macrophages from patients with alpha-1-antitrypsin deficiency spontaneously release the leukocyte chemo-attractant leukotriene B4 [70]. Moreover, in such patients deficiency of a chemotactic factor inactivator has been described [71], which may enhance recruitment of neutrophils to the airspaces in these subjects [72].

Other studies which have suggested that neutrophils from smokers have an enhanced chemotactic activity. Indeed circulating neutrophils from passive cigarette smokers appear to be sensitised to chemotactic signals [73], as do cells from patients with emphysema, compared to age and smoking matched controls [74]. Thus cigarette smoking appears to lead to increased neutrophil sequestration in the lungs and increased chemotactic activity.

4   Evidence of oxidative stress in smokers and patients with COPD.

The evidence for the presence of increased oxidative stress in smokers and patients with COPD is now overwhelming [75-77]. Direct measurements of specific markers of oxidative injury resulting from excessive free radical activity can be made by electron spin resonance, which cannot be applied to the study of tissues at present. Most studies have therefore relied on indirect measurements of free radical activity in biological fluids. Although these markers suggest that oxidative stress has occurred, they do not indicate that this event is necessarily involved in the pathogenesis of the condition which is being studied. Markers of oxidative stress have been shown to occur in the epithelial lining fluid, in the breath and in the urine in cigarette smokers and patients with COPD.

4.1   Antioxidants in bronchoalveolar lavage fluid.

The major antioxidants in RTLF include mucin, reduced glutathione, uric acid, protein (largely albumin) and ascorbic acid [32,78]. Mucin is a glycoprotein rich in cysteine residues (sulphydryls), and hence is an important antioxidant of the RTLF. Mucins have metal binding properties [79], effectively scavenge hydroxyl radical (OH) [80] and would be expected to scavenge OCL^-/HOCL [81] because of the abundance of sulphydryl and disulphide moieties in their structure [82]. Toxic inhalants increase the secretion of mucins, which therefore represent a major antioxidant in the upper RTLFs. However, oxygen radicals are known to degrade mucus glycoproteins [33]. It is therefore likely that cigarette smoke oxidants also react with this respiratory tract secretory glycoprotein.

There is limited information on the respiratory epithelial antioxidant defences in smokers, and less for COPD. Several studies have shown that GSH is elevated in bronchoalveolar lavage fluid (BALF) in the airways of chronic smokers [83,84].

Despite the two-fold increase in BALF GSH in chronic smokers, GSH may not be present in sufficient quantities to deal with the excessive oxidant burden during acute smoking, when acute depletion of GSH may occur [37]. Rahman and colleagues [39,85] studied the acute effects of cigarette smoke condensate (CSC) on GSH metabolism in a human alveolar epithelial cell line *in vitro*, and *in vivo* in rat lungs after intra-tracheal CSC instillation. They found a dose and time-dependent depletion of intracellular GSH, concomitant with the formation of GSH-conjugates, which is supported by similar results in studies in animal lungs *in vivo* [39,85]. Furthermore, the activities of glutathione redox system enzymes, such as glutathione peroxidase and glucose 6-phosphate dehydrogenase, were transiently decreased in alveolar epithelial cells and in rat lungs after CSC exposure, possibly as a result of the action of highly electrophilic free radicals on the active site of the enzymes. GSH homeostasis may also play a central role in the maintenance of the integrity of the lung airspace epithelial barrier. In particular, lowering the levels of GSH in epithelial cells leads to loss of barrier function and increased permeability [38,39].

Pacht and co-workers [86] showed reduced levels of vitamin E in the BAL fluid of smokers compared with non-smokers. By contrast, Bui and colleagues [87] found a marginal increase in vitamin C in BALF of smokers, compared to non-smokers. Similarly, alveolar macrophages from smokers have both increased levels of ascorbic acid and augmented uptake of ascorbate [88]. Enhanced activity of antioxidant enzymes (SOD, and catalase) in alveolar macrophages from young smokers has also been reported [89]. However, Kondo and co-workers [90] found that increased superoxide generation by alveolar macrophages in elderly smokers was associated with decreased antioxidant enzyme activities when compared with non-smokers. The activities of CuZnSOD, glutathione-S-transferase and glutathione peroxidase (GP) were found to be decreased in alveolar macrophages from elderly smokers. This reduced activity was not associated with decreased gene expression, but was due to modification at the post-translational level [90].

The apparent discrepancies between these studies of the levels of the different antioxidants in BALF and alveolar macrophages may be due to different smoking histories in chronic smokers, particularly the time of the last cigarette in relation to the sampling of BALF.

Activities of SOD and GP_x are also higher in the lungs of rats exposed to cigarette smoke [91]. McCusker and Hoidal [89] demonstrated enhanced alveolar macrophage antioxidant enzyme activities following cigarette smoke exposure, which resulted in reduced mortality when the hamsters were subsequently exposed to >95% oxygen. They speculated that mammalian alveolar macrophages undergo an adaptive response to chronic oxidant exposure that may ameliorate the potential damage to lung cells from further oxidant stress. The mechanisms for the induction of antioxidants enzymes in erythrocytes [92], alveolar macrophages [89] and lungs [91] by cigarette smoke exposure are currently unknown. However, it is likely to be due to the induction of antioxidant genes (see below).

Urine isoprostane $F_2\alpha$-III, which is an isomer of prostaglandin, formed by free radical peroxidation of arachidonic acid, has recently been shown to be elevated in patients with COPD, compared with healthy controls, and to be even more elevated in exacerbations of the condition [93].

4.2   Evidence of systemic oxidative stress.

There has recently been considerable interest in the systemic effects of COPD [94]. One manifestation of a systemic effect is the presence of markers of oxidative stress in the blood in patients with COPD. This is reflected in the increased sequestration of neutrophils in the pulmonary microcirculation during smoking and during exacerbations of COPD which, as described above, is an oxidant-mediated event [57,58,75].

Rahman and colleagues [65] demonstrated increased production of superoxide anion from peripheral blood neutrophils obtained from patients with acute exacerbations of COPD, which returned to normal when the patients were restudied when clinically stable. Other studies have shown that circulating neutrophils from patients with COPD have upregulation of their surface adhesion molecules, which may also be an oxidant-mediated effect [95]. Neutrophils activation may be even more pronounced in neutrophils which are sequestered in the pulmonary microcirculation in smokers and in patients with COPD, since animal models of lung inflammation have shown that neutrophils which are sequestered in the pulmonary microcirculation release more reactive oxygen species than circulating neutrophils in the same animal [96]. Thus neutrophils which are sequestered in the pulmonary microcirculation may be a source of oxidative stress, that may have a role in inducing airway injury in COPD, particularly during exacerbations of the condition.

Polyunsaturated fats and fatty acids in cell membranes are a major target of free radical attack, resulting in lipid peroxidation, a process that may continue as a chain reaction to generate peroxides and aldehydes. Products of lipid peroxidation reactions can be measured in body fluids as thiobarbituric acid reactive substances (TBARS). The levels of TBARS in plasma or in bronchoalveolar lavage fluid, are significantly increased in healthy smokers and patients with acute exacerbations of COPD, compared with healthy non-smokers [27,91]. There is however a problem with the specificity of thiobarbituric acid-malondialehyde assays as a measure of lipid peroxidation, since this assay does not directly measure the lipid peroxidation reaction. Other studies have measured conjugated levels of dienes of linoleic acid, a secondary product of lipid peroxidation, and shown the levels in plasma were elevated in chronic smokers [97]. In addition circulating levels of F_2-isoprostane, which is a more direct measurement of lipid peroxidation have been found in smokers [98]. Similarly Lapenna and colleagues [99] demonstrated increased levels of fluorescent products of lipid peroxidation in smokers.

A recent study directly examined the balance between oxidants/antioxidants in smokers and patients with acute exacerbations of COPD by measuring changes in the antioxidant capacity in the blood. Rahman et al [94] found that the plasma antioxidant capacity was significantly decreased in smokers 1 hour after smoking and in patients with acute exacerbations of COPD, when compared with plasma from age- matched non-smoking controls. The decrease in plasma antioxidant capacity in smokers may be due to a profound depletion of plasma protein sulphydryls as demonstrated following cigarette smoke exposure *in vitro* [100-102]. Thus there is clear evidence that oxidants in cigarette smoke markedly decrease low molecular plasma antioxidants both *in vitro* and *in vivo*. Depletion of plasma antioxidants reduces the protection against cigarette smoke-induced plasma membrane peroxidation. It is possible that individual variations in the ability to enhance the antioxidant screen in body fluids may be one factor which accounts for the susceptibility of some smokers to develop COPD.

Likewise, investigators have measured the major plasma antioxidants in smokers [103-109]. These studies show a depletion of ascorbic acid vitamin E, β-carotene and selenium in the serum of chronic smokers [104,105,107-109]. Moreover, decreased vitamin E and vitamin C levels were measured in leukocytes from smokers [110-113]. However, circulating red blood cells from cigarette smokers contain increased levels of SOD and catalase, despite similar activity of glutathione peroxidase, and are better able to protect endothelial cells from the effects of H_2O_2, when compared with cells from non-smokers [92].

Plasma ascorbate may be a particularly important antioxidant in the plasma because the gas phase of cigarette smoke induces lipid peroxidation in plasma *in vitro* that is decreased by ascorbate [114]. Inhalation of NO from cigarette smoke, as well as NO and superoxide anion released by activated phagocytes react to form peroxynitrite which is cytotoxic. Peroxynitrite has recently been shown to decrease plasma antioxidant capacity, by rapid oxidation of ascorbic acid, uric acid and plasma sulphydryls [115]. Evidence of NO/peroxynitrite activity in plasma has been demonstrated in cigarette smokers. Nitration of tyrosine residues or proteins in plasma leads to the production of 3-nitrotyrosine. Petiuzzelli and colleagues [116] demonstrated the presence of 3-nitrotyrosine in plasma in smokers, which were present in higher levels than in a small group of non-smokers. They also confirmed low levels of antioxidant capacity in smokers [94], which were negatively correlated with the levels of 3-nitrotyrosine [116]. The levels of antioxidant capacity in the plasma has a negative correlation with the increased release of oxygen radicals, from circulating neutrophils in patients with exacerbations of COPD [94].

5   Other mechanisms related to the pathogenesis of COPD involving oxidants.

The majority of the information which is available on the pathogenesis of COPD relates to the development of emphysema. COPD also encompasses the conditions chronic bronchitis and chronic bronchiolitis. It is presumed that the mechanisms which initiate inflammation and the effects of proteolytic and oxidant-induced damage are also relevant to these conditions, although much less information is available.

Animal models of elastase induced emphysema also show features of airways diseases with goblet cells hyperplasia [117]. Neutrophil elastase is known to be a potent secretagog for mucous glands and therefore may contribute to the hyper-mucous secretion in chronic bronchitis [118]. Oxidant generated systems, such as Xanthine/Xanthine oxidase have also been shown to cause the release of mucous [119]. Both oxidants and neutrophil elastase can injure airway epithelial cells [120,121].

6   Oxidant / antioxidant balance and the development of airways obstruction.

The neutrophil appears to be a critical cell in the pathogenesis of COPD. Previous epidemiological studies have shown a relationship between circulating neutrophil numbers and the FEV_1 [122]. Other studies have provided supportive evidence of a role for reactive oxygen species released from circulating neutrophils and the development of airflow limitation. Richards et al have shown a relationship between peripheral blood neutrophil chemiluminescence and measures of airflow limitation in young cigarette smokers [123]. Even passive cigarette smoking has been associated with increased peripheral blood leukocyte counts and enhanced release of oxygen radicals [124]. Oxidative stress, measured as TBARS in plasma has also been shown to correlate inversely with the % predicted FEV_1 in a population study, indicating that lipid peroxidation is associated with airflow limitation [125].

In the general population an association between dietary intake of antioxidant vitamins and lung function has been demonstrated. Britton and co-workers [126]. In a population of 2,633 subjects they showed an association between dietary intake of the antioxidant vitamin E and lung function, supporting the hypothesis that this antioxidant may have a role in protecting against the development of COPD. This study supports the concept that vitamin supplementation may be a possible preventive therapy against the development of COPD. Such intervention studies have been difficult to carry out [127], but there is at least some evidence to suggest that antioxidant vitamin supplementation reduces oxidant stress, measured as a decrease in Pentane levels in breath as an assessment of lipid peroxides [128].

7   Oxidative stress and gene expression.

7.1   Pro-inflammatory genes.

There is overwhelming evidence that COPD is associated with airway and airspace inflammation, as shown for example by recent biopsy studies [129]. Numerous markers of inflammation have been shown to be elevated in the sputum of patients with COPD, including IL-8 and TNFα [130].

Genes for many inflammatory mediators, such as the cytokines, IL-8, TNFα, and nitric oxide are regulated by transcription factors such as nuclear factor kappa B (NF-κB). NF-κB is present in the cytosol in an inactive form linked to its inhibitory protein IκB. Many stimuli, including cytokines and oxidants, activate NF-κB, resulting in ubiquination, cleaving of IκB from NF-κB and the destruction of IκB in the proteozome [131]. This critical event in the inflammatory response is redox sensitive. We have shown in preliminary studies *in vitro* using both macrophage cell lines and alveolar and bronchial epithelial cells, that oxidants cause the release of inflammatory mediators such as IL-8, IL-1, and nitric oxide and that these events are associated with increased expression of the genes for these inflammatory mediators and increased nuclear binding or activation of NF-κB [132,133]. We have also shown that stimuli relevant to the development to exacerbations of COPD, such as particulate air pollution which has oxidant properties also activates NF-κB in alveolar epithelial cells [134].

Thiol antioxidants such as N-acetylcysteine and Nacystelin, which have potential as therapies in COPD, have been shown in *in vitro* experiments to block the release of these inflammatory mediators from epithelial cells and macrophages, by a mechanism involving increasing intracellular glutathione and decreased NF-κB activation [132,133].

7.2   Antioxidant genes.

As described above there is considerable evidence for an increased oxidant burden in the lungs of smokers and patients with COPD. An important effect of oxidative stress is the upregulation of protective antioxidant genes. The antioxidant glutathione is concentrated in epithelial lining fluid compared with plasma [78] and appears to have an important protective role, together with its redox enzymes in the airspaces and intracellularly in epithelial cells. To illustrate the protective role of glutathione against the effects of cigarette smoke we have developed models *in vivo* in the rat and *in vitro* using monolayer cultures of alveolar epithelial cells, to assess the injurious effects of cigarette smoke. Human studies have shown that glutathione is elevated in epithelial lining fluid in chronic cigarette smokers, compared with non-smokers, an increase which does not occur during acute cigarette smoking [27]. The effects of acute and chronic cigarette smoking can be mimicked following intratracheal instillation of cigarette smoke condensate in the rat and exposure of epithelial cell monolayers to cigarette smoke *in vitro* [37,85,135]. Following exposure to cigarette smoke there is a profound decrease in GSH in BAL in the rat that is mirrored by a fall in total lung GSH 6 hours after exposure [75,135]. Similarly there is a fall in intracellular GSH in epithelial cells following exposure to cigarette smoke condensate [37,85]. There is an association between the fall in lung and intracellular glutathione both *in vivo* and *in vitro* and an increase in epithelial permeability, as described above.

We have used a rat model of intratracheal instillation of cigarette smoke condensate *in vivo* and exposure of epithelial cell monolayers *in vitro* to study the regulation of glutathione and its redox system in response to cigarette smoke condensate and other oxidants, and in particular to investigate the discrepancy between glutathione levels in chronic and acute cigarette smoking. Following exposure of airspace epithelial cells to cigarette smoke condensate *in vitro* there is an initial decrease in intracellular GSH, with a rebound increase when the cells are washed and culture is continued for 24 hours [136]. This effect *in vitro* was mimicked by a similar change in glutathione in rat lungs *in vivo* following intratracheal instillation of cigarette smoke condensate [85], associated with an increase in the oxidised form (GSSG). We also examined the activity of the major enzymes involved in glutathione synthesis and in the glutathione redox system in response to cigarette smoke condensate both *in vivo* and *in vitro*. The initial fall in lung and intracellular glutathione after treatment with cigarette smoke condensate was associated with decreased activity of γGCS the rate limiting enzyme of glutathione synthesis, with recovery of the activity by 24 hours [85,136]. We hypothesise that the increased levels of glutathione following cigarette smoke condensate exposure may be due to induction of the γGCS gene by components within cigarette smoke. Using reverse transcriptase polymerase chain reaction we showed an increase in γ-GCS mRNA expression 12-24 hours after airspace epithelial cells were exposed to cigarette smoke condensate *in vitro* [136,137] (Figure 3). We also demonstrated that the upregulation of γGCS gene expression occurred at the transcriptional level. We suggested that this might be due to activation of redox-sensitive transcription factors involved in the regulation of γGCS expression. In a series of experiments using both the gel mobility shift assay and reporter system in which the promoter region of γGCS gene was transfected into airway epithelial cells, we showed that cigarette smoke condensate activated the transcription factor activator protein-1 (AP-1) [138,139]. In deletion experiments and using site- directed mutagenisis in a promoter system we demonstrated that a proximal AP-1 is critical for the regulation of γ-glutamylcysteine synthetase gene expression in response to various oxidants including cigarette smoke (Figure 4) [138] and hence glutathione synthesis in lung epithelial cells. Thus oxidative stress, including that produced by cigarette smoking, causes upregulation of an important gene involved in the synthesis of glutathione as an adaptive or protective effect against oxidative stress. These events are likely to account for the increased glutathione levels seen in the epithelial lining fluid in chronic cigarette smokers, which acts as a protective mechanism. The injurious effects of cigarette smoke may occur repeatedly during and immediately after cigarette smoking when the lung is depleted of antioxidants including glutathione. The cytokine tumour necrosis factor (TNF), which is thought to have a role in the lung inflammation in COPD also decreases intracellular glutathione levels initially, in epithelial cells, by a mechanism involving intra-cellular oxidative stress, which is followed 12-24 hours thereafter by a rebound increase in intracellular glutathione as a result of AP-1 activation and an increased γGCS expression [137]. Corticosteroids have been used as anti-inflammatory agents in COPD, but there is still doubt over their effectiveness in reducing airway inflammation in COPD. Interestingly dexamethasone also causes a decrease in intracellular glutathione in airspace epithelial cells, but no rebound increase, compared with the effects of TNF [137]. Moreover, the rebound increase in glutathione produced by TNF in epithelial cells is prevented by co-treatment with dexamethasone [137]. These effects may have relevance for the treatment of COPD patients with corticosteroids.

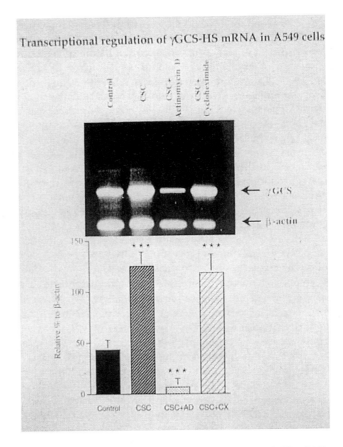

Figure 3. Effect of cigarette smoke on gamma-glutamylcysteine synthetase (γGCS) mRNA expression in alveolar epithelial cells (A549) exposed to cigarette smoke condensate (CSC). The upper panel shows γGCS gene expression by RTPCR which increases following exposure to CSC. This effect was blocked by actinomycin D (AD) but not by cycloheximide (CX). The lower panel shows the densitometry of the γGCS band relative to β-actin. These results show that cigarette smoke increases the expression of γGCS mRNA in alveolar epithelial cells, an effect which is at the transcriptional level.

Recently Gilks and co-workers [140] have shown increased expression of a number of antioxidant genes in the bronchial epithelial cells in rats exposed to whole cigarette smoke for up to 14 days. Whereas mRNA of manganese superoxide dismutase (MnSOD) and metallothioneine (MT) was increased at 1-2 days and returned to normal by 7 days, mRNA for glutathione peroxidase did not increased until 7 days exposure, suggesting the importance of the glutathione redox system as a mechanism for chronic protection against the effects of cigarette smoke [140].

The *c-fos* gene belongs to a family of growth and differentiation-related immediate early genes, the expression of which generally represents the first measurable response to a variety of chemical and physical stimuli [131]. Studies in various cell lines have shown enhanced gene expression of *c-fos* in response to cigarette smoke condensate [141,142]. These effects of cigarette smoke condensate can be mimicked by peroxynitrite and smoke-related aldehydes in concentrations that are present in cigarette smoke condensate [141]. The effects of cigarette smoke condensate can be enhanced by pre-treatment of the cells with buthionine sulfoxamine to decrease intracellular glutathione and can be prevented by treatment with N-acetylcysteine, a thiol antioxidant [141]. These studies emphasise the importance, of intracellular levels of the antioxidant glutathione in gene expression.

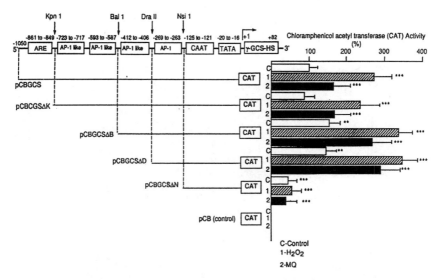

Figure 4. The 5'-flanking successive deletion sequence of the γ-GCS-HS gene from oligonucleotides -1050, -818, -511, -305, -201 to $+82$ bp were cloned into pCAT-Basic and co-transfected into A549 alveolar epithelial cells along with the control plasmid PSV-β-Gal. Panel A shows the relative positions of the *cis*-acting DNA elements and a restriction map of the promoter region cloned in pCRII vector. The numbers in the figure represent the nucleotide positions from the transcriptional start site of the γ-GCS-HS gene, which is indicated by the bent arrow on the right. The dotted line on the left indicates an additional 50bp from multiple cloning sites of the pCRII vector. The structure of the γ-GCS-HS CAT plasmids are shown below on the right. Deletion mutants were ligated to upstream of the CAT gene in pCAT Basic vector (pCB) and its constitutive transcriptional CAT activity was measured 36-48 h post-transfection. Various deleted constructs were transfected into A549 cells and exposed to H_2O_2 (100 μM) and MQ (100 μM). After 24 h incubation, the cells were harvested and assayed for CAT activity. Panel B: Transcriptional activity among different constructs was standardised by the amount of CAT activity relative to β-Gal activity. The results are shown as percentages of the CAT concentration compared to that of pCBGCS. Each histogram represents the mean and the bars the SEM of four independent transfections, each performed in duplicate with the activity pCBGCS set at 100%. **$p<0.01$, ***$p<0.001$, compared to pCBGCS.

Thus oxidative stress, including that produced by cigarette smoke, causes increased gene expression of both injurious pro-inflammatory genes by oxidant- mediated activation of transcription factors such as NFκB, but also activation of protective genes such as γ-glutamylcysteine synthetase through other transcription factors, which in the case of γ-GCS is the transcription factor AP-1. A balance may therefore exist between pro and "anti-inflammatory" gene expression in response to cigarette smoke, which may be critical to whether cell injury is induced by cigarette smoking (Figure 5). Knowledge of the molecular mechanisms that regulate these events may open new therapeutic avenues in the treatment of COPD.

8   Oxidative stress and susceptibility to COPD.

It is well recognised that since only a proportion — 15-20% of cigarette smokers appear to be susceptible to its effects, show a rapid decline in FEV_1 and develop the disease [143], there has been considerable interest in identifying those who are most susceptible and the mechanisms of that susceptibility [143,144], since this would provide an important insight into the pathogenesis of COPD as did the recognition of an association between α_1-antitrypsin and COPD [145].

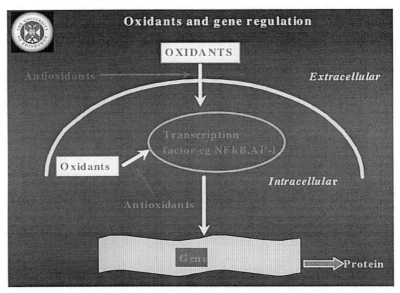

Figure 5. The effect of oxidants on intracellular GSH redox status and NF-κB and AP-1 nuclear translocation. Oxidants cause nuclear translocation of NF-κB which upregulates genes for cytokines such as TNF and IL-1 which themselves can produce oxidative stress through the release of oxidants from mitochondrial electron transfer chain which may result in decreased intracellular GSH. In addition oxidants can upregulate AP-1 which can cause nuclear translocation of AP-1 which has been shown to increase messenger RNA for γGCS which will increase intracellular glutathione. An imbalance may develop between these pro and anti-inflammatory effects of oxidant-mediated gene regulation.

Severe α_1-antitrypsin deficiency is the only proven genetic risk factor for COPD. Studies of relatives of patients who develop severe early onset COPD and who do not have α_1-antitrypsin deficiency, had an increase risk of the development of COPD compared to relatives of subjects who did not have the disease.

Polymorphisms of various genes have been shown to be more prevalent in smokers who develop COPD than in non-smokers [144]. A number of these polymorphisms may have functional significance, such as the association between the TNF α gene polymorphism (TNF2) which may be associated with increased TNF levels in response to inflammation, and the development of chronic bronchitis [145]. Relevant to the effects of cigarette smoke is a polymorphism in the gene for microsomal epoxide hydrolase, which is an enzyme involved in the metabolism of highly reactive epoxide intermediates which are present in cigarette smoke [146]. The proportion of individuals with a slow microsomal epoxide hydrolase activity (homozygoes) was significantly higher in patients with COPD and in a subgroup of patients shown pathologically to have emphysema (COPD 22%;

emphysema 19%) compared with control subjects (6%). It may be that a panel of the "susceptibility" polymorphisms, of functional significance in enzymes involved in xenobiotic metabolism or antioxidant enzyme genes may allow individuals to be identified as being susceptible to the effects of cigarette smoke.

9   Therapeutic options for redressing the oxidant/antioxidant imbalance in COPD

Having demonstrated evidence for an oxidant/antioxidant imbalance in smokers and its probable role in the pathogenesis of COPD do we have any therapeutic options? Various approaches have been tried to redress this imbalance. One approach would be to target the inflammatory response by reducing the sequestration or migration of leukocytes from the pulmonary circulation into the airspaces. Possible therapeutic options for this are drugs that alter cell deformability, so preventing neutrophil sequestration or the migration of neutrophils, either by interfering with adhesion molecules necessary for migration, or preventing the release of inflammatory cytokines such as IL-8 or leukotriene B4 which result in neutrophil migration. It should also be possible to use anti-inflammatory agents to prevent the release of oxygen radicals from activated leukocytes or to quench those oxidants once they are formed, by enhancing the antioxidant screen in the lungs.

There are various options to enhance the lung antioxidant screen. One approach would be the molecular manipulation of antioxidant genes, such as glutathione peroxidase or genes involved in the synthesis of glutathione, such as γGCS or by developing molecules with activity similar to those of antioxidants enzymes such as catalase and superoxide dismutase. Another approach would simply be to administer antioxidant therapy. This has been attempted in cigarette smokers using various antioxidants such as vitamin C and vitamin E [147-150]. The results have been rather disappointing, although as described above the antioxidant vitamin E has been shown to reduce oxidative stress in patients with COPD [128]. Attempts to supplement lung glutathione have been tried using the glutathione or its precursors [151]. Glutathione itself is not efficiently transported into most animal cells and an excess of glutathione may be a source of the thiol radical under conditions of oxidative stress [152]. Nebulised glutathione has also been used therapeutically but this has been shown to induce bronchial hyperreactivity [153]. Cysteine is a thiol that is the rate limiting amino acid in GSH synthesis [154]. Cysteine administration is not possible since it is oxidised to cystine that is neurotoxic [155]. The cysteine donating compound N-acetylcysteine (NAC) acts as a cellular precursor of GSH and becomes de-acetylated in the gut to cysteine following oral administration. It reduces disulphide bonds and has the potential to interact directly with oxidants. The use of N-acetylcysteine in an attempt to enhance GSH in patients with COPD has met with varying success [156,157]. NAC given orally in low doses of 600 mgs per day to normal subjects results in very low levels of NAC in the plasma for up to 2 hours after administration [156]. Bridgeman and colleagues [157] showed after 5 days of NAC 600 mg 3 times daily, that there was a significant increase in plasma GSH levels. However, there was no associated rise in BAL GSH nor GSH in lung tissue. These data seem to imply that producing a sustained increase in lung GSH is difficult using NAC in subjects who are not already depleted of glutathione. In spite of this continental European studies have shown that NAC reduces the number of exacerbation days in patients with COPD [158,159]. This was not confirmed in a British Thoracic Society study of NAC [160]. The contradictory results of these studies may result from several reasons; firstly the positive studies of NAC were in patients who had relatively mild COPD, whereas in the British Study the patients had more severe COPD. Secondly, relatively small doses of N-acetylcysteine was given in both studies.

N-acystelyn (NAL) is a lysine salt of N-acetylinecysteine. It is also a mucolytic and oxidant thiol compound which in contrast to NAC which is acid, has a neutral pH. NAL can be given by inhalation into the lung without causing significant side effects [161]. Studies comparing the effects of NAL and NAC found that both drugs enhanced intracellular glutathione in alveolar epithelial cells [162] and inhibited hydrogen peroxide and superoxide anion release from neutrophils harvested from peripheral blood from smokers and patients with COPD [162].

Most animal cells normally export glutathione, and do not take up intact Glutathione. glutathione ethyl ester contains an ethyl group that is esterified to the glycine of glutathione. Glutathione ethyl ester is more lipophylic and thus passes more readily into cells than glutathione. The monoester is then hydrolysed to glutathione by cytosolic non-specific esterase [163]. Glutathione monoethyl ester is resistant to the cleavage by the enzyme γ-glutamylcysteine transpeptidase and has been used to increase glutathione *in vitro* [164]. Thiazolidine is a potentially useful compound for cysteine delivery and can be shown to protect against oxidative injury [165]. However, there are no studies in humans which validate these compounds for clinical trials.

OXIDANT-MEDIATED LUNG INJURY IN SMOKERS

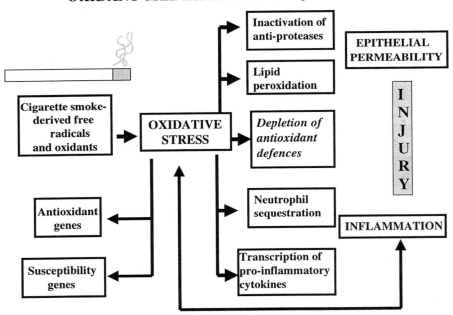

Figure 6. Oxidant mediated lung injury in smokers.

Molecular regulation of glutathione synthesis, by targeting γGCS has great promise as a means of treating oxidant medicated injury in the lungs. Cellular GSH may be increased by increasing γGCS activity. This may be possible by gene transfer techniques, although this would be an expensive treatment that may not be considered for a condition such as COPD. However, knowledge of how γGCS is regulated may allow the development of other compounds that may act to enhance GSH.

In summary, there is now very good evidence for an oxidant/antioxidant imbalance in COPD and increasing evidence that this imbalance is important in the pathogenesis of this condition. There are a number of important effects of oxidative stress in smokers that are relevant to the development of COPD (Figure 6). Oxidative stress may also be critical to the inflammatory response to cigarette smoke, through the upregulation of redox-sensitive transcription factors and hence pro-inflammatory gene expression; but is also involved in the protective mechanisms against the effects of cigarette smoke by the induction of antioxidant genes. Inflammation itself induces oxidative stress in the lungs and polymorphisms on genes for inflammatory mediators or antioxidant genes may have a role in the susceptibility to the effects of cigarette smoke.

Knowledge of the mechanisms of the effects of oxidative stress should in future allow the development of potent antioxidant therapies which test the hypothesis that oxidative stress is involved in the pathogenesis of COPD, not only by direct injury to cells, but also as a fundamental factor in inflammation in smoking-related lung disease.

References.

1.   Murray CJL, Lopez AD. (1997) Mortality by cause for eight regions of the world : global burden of disease study. *Lancet*;**349**:1269-1276.
2.   Standards of Care Committee of the British Thoracic Society. (1997) BTS Guidelines for the management of chronic obstructive pulmonary disease. *Thorax*;**52** (Suppl 5):S1-S28.
3.   Church T, Pryor WA. (1985) Free-radical chemistry of cigarette smoke and its toxicological implications. *Environ. Health Perspect.*;**64**:111-26.
4.   Rahman I, MacNee W. (1996) Role of oxidants/antioxidants in smoking-induced lung diseases. *Free Rad. Biol. Med.*;**21**:669-681.
5.   Taylor JC, Kueppers F. (1977) Electrophoretic mobility of leukocyte elastase of normal subjects and patients with chronic obstructive pulmonary disease. *Am. Rev. Respir. Dis.*;**116**:531-536.
6.   Kramps JA, Bakker W, Dihkman JH. (1980) A matched-pair study of the leukocyte elastase-like activity in normal persons and in emphysematous patients with and without alpha-1-antitrypsin deficiency. *Am. Rev. Respir. Dis.*;**121**:253-261.
7.   Burnett D, Chamba A, Hill SL, Stockley RA. (1987) Neutrophils from subjects with chronic obstructive lung disease show enhanced chemotaxis and extracellular proteolysis. *Lancet*;**ii**:1043-1046.
8.   Hubbard R, McElvaney N, Crystal RG. Amount of neutrophil elastase carried by neutrophils may modulate the extent of emphysema in ∝-1-antitrypsin deficiency. *Am. Rev. Respir. Dis.* 10990;**141**:A682.
9.   Chamba A, Afford SC, Stockley RA, Burnett D. (1991) Extracellular proteolysis of fibronectin by neutrophils: characterization and the effects of recombinant cytokines. *Am. J. Respir. Cell Moll. Biol.*;**4**:330-337.
10.   Gadek J, Fells GA, Crystal RG. Cigarette smoking induces functional antiprotease deficiency in the lower respiratory tract of humans. *Science* 1979;**206**:1315-1316.
11.   Carp H, Janoff A. (1980) Inactivation of bronchial mucous proteinase inhibitor by cigarette smoke and phagocyte-derived oxidants. *Exp. Lung Res.*;**1**:225-237.
12.   Hubbard RC, Ogushi F, Fels GA, Cantin AM, Courtney M Crystal RG. (1987) Oxidants spontaneously released by alveolar macrophages of cigarette smokers can inactivate the active site of alpha 1-antitrypsin rendering it ineffective as an inhibitor of neutrophil elastase. *J. Clin. Invest.*;**80**:1289-95.
13.   Kramps JA, Rudolphus A, Stolk J, Willems LNA, Dijkman JH, (1991) Role of antileukoprotease in the lung. *Ann. N. Y. Acad. Sci., USA.*;**624**:97-108.
14.   Kramps JA, van Twisk C, Dijkman DH. (1988) Oxidative inactivation of antileukoprotease is triggered by polymorphonuclear leukocytes. *Clin Sci*;**75**:53-62.
15.   Johnson D, Travis J. (1979) The oxidative inactivation of human ∝1-proteinase inhibitor. Further evidence for methionine at the reactive center *J. Biol. Chem.*;**254**:4022-4026.
16.   Carp H, Janoff A. (1978) Possible mechanisms of emphysema in smokers: in vitro suppression of serum elastase-inhibitory capacity by fresh cigarette smoke and its prevention by anti-oxidants. *Am. Rev. Respir. Dis.*;**118**:617-621.

17.   Carp H, Miller F, Hoidal JR, Janoff A. (1982) Potential mechanisms of emphysema: ∝1-proteinase inhibitor recovered from lungs of cigarette smokers contains oxidised methionine and has decreased elastase inhibitory capacity. *Proc. Natl. Acad. Sci.*;**79:** 2041-2045.

18.   Janoff A, Carp H, Laurent P, Raju L. (1983) The role of oxidative processes in emphysema. *Am. Rev. Respir. Dis.*;**127:**S31-S38.

19.   Stone P, Calore JD, McGowan SE *et al* (1983). Functional alpha-1-protease inhibitor in the lower respiratory tract of smokers is not decreased. *Science*;**221:**1187-1189.

20.   Afford SC, Burnett D, Campbell EJ *et al.* (1988) The assessment of ∝-1-proteinase inhibitor form and function in lung lavage fluid from healthy subjects. *Biol. Chem. Hoppe Seyler*;**369:**1065-1074.

21.   Abboud RT, Fera T, Richter A *et al.* (1985) Acute effect of smoking on the functional activity of alpha-1-protease inhibitor in bronchoalveolar lavage fluid. *Am. Rev. Respir. Dis.*;**131:**1187-1189.

22.   Ogushi F, Hubbard RC, Vogelmeier C *et al.* (1991) Risk factors for emphysema. Cigarette smoking is associated with a reduction in the association rate constant of lung ∝1-antitrypsin for neutrophil elastase. *J. Clin. Invest.*;**87:**1060-1065.

23.   Bluhm AC, Weistein J, Sonsa JA. (1971) Free radicals in tobacco smoke. *Nature*;**229:**500

24.   Pryor WA, Stone K. (1993) Oxidants in cigarette smoke: radicals hydrogen peroxides peroxynitrate and peroxynitrite. *Annals N. Y. Acad. Sci.*;**686:**12-28.

25.   Nakayama T, Church DF, Pryor WA. Quantitative analysis of the hydrogen peroxide formed in aqueous cigarette tar extracts. *Free Rad. Biol. Med.* 1989;7:9-15.

26.   Hunninghake GW, Crystal RG. (1983) Cigarette smoking and lung destruction : Accumulation of neutrophils in the lungs of cigarette smokers. *Am. Rev. Respir. Dis.*;**128:**833-838.

27.   Morrison D, Rahman I, Lannan S, MacNee W. (1999) Epithelial permeability inflammation and oxidant stress in the air spaces of smokers. *Am. J. Respir. Crit. Care Med.*;**159:**473-479.

28.   Mateos F, Brock JF, Perez-Arellano JL. (1998) Iron metabolism in the lower respiratory tract, *Thorax*;**53:**594-600.

29.   Thompson AB, Bohling T, Heires A, Linder J, Rennard SI. (1991) Lower respiratory tract iron burden is increased in association with cigarette smoking. *J Lab. Clin. Med.*;**117:**494-499.

30.   Wesselius LJ, Nelson ME, Skikne BS. (1994) Increased release of ferritin and iron by iron loaded alveolar macrophages in cigarette smokers. *Am. J. Respir. Crit. Care Med*;**150:**690-695.

31.   Laurent P, Janoff A, Kagan HM. (1983) Cigarette smoke blocks cross-linking of elastin in vitro. *Am. Rev. Respir. Dis*;**127:**189-192.

32.   Cross CE, Van der Vliet A, O'Neill CA, Louie S, Halliwell B. (1994) Oxidants antioxidants and respiratory tract lining fluids. *Environ. Health Perspect.*;**102** (Suppl 10):185-191.

33.   Cross CE, Halliwell B, Allen A. (1984) Antioxidant protection : a function of tracheobranchial and gastrointestinal mucus. *Lancet*;**1:**1328-1330.

34.   Dye JA, Adler KB. (1994) Effects of cigarette smoke on epithelial cells on the respiratory tract. *Thorax*;**49:**825-834.

35.   Jones JG, Lawler P, Crawley JCW, Minty BD, Hulands G, Veall N. (1981) Increased alveolar epithelial permeability in cigarette smokers. *Lancet*:66-68.

36.   Lannan S, Donaldson K, Brown D, MacNee W. (1994) Effects of cigarette smoke and its condensates on alveolar cell injury in vitro. *Am. J. Physiol.*;**266:**L92-L100.

37.   Li XY, Donaldson K, Rahman I, MacNee W. (1994) An investigation of the role of glutathione in the increased epithelial permeability induced by cigarette smoke in vivo and in vitro. *Am. J. Respir. Crit. Care Med*;**149:**1518-1525.

38.   Li XY, Rahman I, Donaldson K, MacNee W. (1999) Mechanisms of cigarette smoke induced increased airspace permeability. *Thorax* in press

39.   Rahman I, Li XY, Donaldson K, MacNee W. (1995) Cigarette smoke glutathione metabolism and epithelial permeability in rat lungs. *Biochem. Soc. Trans.*;**23:**235S.

40.   Li XY, Donaldson K, Brown D, MacNee W. (1995) The role of tumour necrosis factor in increased airspace epithelial permeability in acute lung inflammation. *Am. J. Resp. Cell Moll. Biol.*;**13:**185-195.

41.   Kilburn K, McKenzie W. (1975) Leukocyte recruitment to airways by cigarette smoke and particle phase in contrast to cytotoxicity of vapour. *Science*;**189:**634-637.

42.   Hunninghake GW, Crystal RG. (1983) Cigarette smoking and lung destruction : Accumulation of neutrophils in the lungs of cigarette smokers. *Am. Rev. Respir. Dis.*;**128:**833-838.

43.   Schaberg T, Haller H, Rau M, Kaiser D, Fassbender M, Lode H. (1992) Superoxide anion release induced by platelet-activating factor is increased in human alveolar macrophages from smokers. *Eur. Respir. J.*;**5:**387-393.

44.   Richards GA, Therson AJ, Carel A, Merwe VD, (1989) Anderson R. Spirometric abnormalities in young smokers correlate with increased chemiluminescence responses of activated blood phagocytes. *Am. Rev. Respir. Dis.*;**139:**181-187.

45. Davis WB, Pacht ER, Spatafora M, Marin WJ II. (1988) Enhanced cytotoxic potential of alveolar macrophages from cigarette smokers. *J. Lab. Clin. Med.*;**111**:293-298.

46. Ludwig PW, Hoidal JR. (1982) Alterations in leukocyte oxidative metabolism in cigarette smokers. *Am. Rev. Respir. Dis.*;**126**:977-980.

47. Hoidal JR, Fox RB, LeMarbe PA, Perri R, Repine JE. (1981) Altered oxidative metabolic responses in vitro of alveolar macrophages from asymptomatic cigarette smokers. *Am. Rev. Respir. Dis.*;**123**:85-89.

48. Bridges RB, Fu MC, Rehm SR. (1985) Increased neutrophil myeloperoxidase activity associated with cigarette smoking. *Eur. J. Respir. Dis*;**67**:84-93.

49. Van Antwerpen VL, Theron AJ, Richards GA, Steenkamp KJ, Van der Merwe CA, Van der Walt R, Anderson R. (1995) Vitamin E pulmonary functions and phagocyte-mediated oxidative stress in smokers and non-smokers *Free Rad. Biol. Med.*;**18**:935-943.

50. Di Stefano A, Capelli A, Lusuardi M, Balbo P, Vecchio C, Maestrelli P, Mapp CE, Fabbri LM, Donner CF, Saetta M. (1998) Severity of airflow limitation is associated with severity of airway inflammation in smokers. *Am. J. Respir. Crit. Care Med.;***158**:1277-1285.

51. Dekhuijzen RPN, Aben KKH, Dekker I, Aarts PHJ, Wielders PML, Van Herwaaden LA Bast A. (1996) Increased exhalation of hydrogen peroxide in patients with stable and unstable chronic obstructive pulmonary disease. *Am. J. Respir. Crit. Care Med.*;**154**:813-816.

52. Maziak W, Loukides S, Culpitt S, Sullivan P, Kharitonov SA, Barnes PJ. (1998) Exhaled nitric oxide in chronic obstructive pulmonary disease. *Am. J. Respir. Crit. Care Med.*;**157**:998-1002.

53. Hoidal JR, Fox RB, LeMarbe PA, Perri R, Repine JE. (1981) Altered oxidative metabolic responses in vitro of alveolar macrophages from asymptomatic cigarette smokers. *Am. Rev. Respir. Dis.*;**123**:85-89.

54. Pinamonti S, Muzzuli M, Chicca C, Papi A, Ravenna F Faabri FM, Ciaccia A. (1996) Xanthine oxidase activity in bronchoalveolar lavage fluid from patients with chronic obstructive lung disease. *Free Radical Biol. Med.*;**21**:147-155.

55. Selby C, MacNee W. (1993) Factors affecting neutrophil transit during acute pulmonary inflammation: minireview. *Exp. Lung Res.*;**19**:407-428.

56. Hogg JC. (1987) Neutrophil kinetics and lung injury. Physiol Rev;**67**:1249-1295.

57. Selby C, Drost E, Lannan S, Wraith PK, MacNee W. (1991) Neutrophil retention in the lungs of patients with chronic obstructive pulmonary diseases. *Am. Rev. Respir. Dis.*;**143**:1359-64.

58. MacNee W, Wiggs B, Berzberg AS, Hogg JC. (1989) The effects of cigarette smoking on neutrophil kinetics in human lungs. *N. Engl. J. Med.*;**321**:924-928.

59. Drost EM, Selby C, Lannan S, Lowe GDO, MacNee W. (1992) Changes in neutrophil deformability following in vitro smoke exposure : mechanism and protection. *Am. J. Respir. Cell Moll. Biol.*;**6**:287-95.

60. Drost EM, Selby C, Bridgeman MME, MacNee W. (1993) Decreased leukocyte deformability after acute cigarette smoking in humans. *Am. Rev. Respir. Dis.*;**148**:1277-1283.

61. Lehr HA, Kress E, Menger MD, Friedl HP, Hubner C, Arfors KE, Messmer K. (1993) Cigarette smoke elicits leukocyte adhesion to endothelium in hamsters : inhibition by CuZnSOD. *Free Rad. Biol. Med.*;**14**:573-581

62. Klut ME, Doerschuk CM, Hogg JC, (1993) Vaneedon SF, Burns AR. Activation of neutrophils within pulmonary microvessels of rabbits exposed to cigarette smoke. *Am. J. Respir. Cell Moll Biol.*;**9**:82-90.

63. Nathan C, Srimal S, Farber C, Sanchez E, Kabbash L, Asch A, Gailit J, Wright S. (1989) Cytokine-induced respiratory burst of human neutrophils dependence on extracellular matrix proteins and CD11/CD18 integrins. *J. Cell Biol.*;**109**:1341-1349.

64. Selby C, Drost E, Brown D, Howie S, MacNee W. (1992) Inhibition of neutrophil adherence and movement by acute cigarette smoke exposure. *Exp. Lung Res.*;**18**:813-827.

65. Rahman I, Skwarska E, MacNee W. (1997) Attenuation of oxidant/antioxidant imbalance during treatment of exacerbations of chronic obstructive pulmonary disease. *Thorax*;**52**:565-568.

66. Totti N, McCusker RT, Campbell EJ *et al.* (1984) Nicotine is chemotactic for neutrophils and enhances neutrophil responsiveness to chemotactic peptides. *Science*;**223**:169-171.

67. Nishikawa M, Kakemizu N, Ito T, Kudo M, Kaneko T, Susuki M, Udaka N, Ikeda H, Okubo T. (1999) Superoxide mediates cigarette smoke-induced infiltration of neutrophils into the airways through nuclear factor-κB activation and IL-8 mRNA expression in guinea pigs in vivo. *Am. J. Respir. Cell Moll. Biol.*;**20**:189-198.

68. Morrison D, Strieter RM, Donnelly SC, Burdick MD, Kunkel SL, MacNee W. (1998) Neutrophil chemokines in bronchoalveolar lavage fluid and leukocyte-conditioned medium from non-smokers and smokers. *Eur. Respir. J.*;**12**:1067-1072.

69. Mills PR, Sapsford RJ, Seemungal T, Develia JL, Davies RJ. (1998) IL-8 release from cultured human bronchial epithelial cells (HBEC) of non-smokers, smokers with normal pulmonary function,

and patients with COPD, and the effect of exposure to diesel exhaust particles (DEP). *Am. J. Respir. Crit. Care Med.*;**157**:A743.

70. Hubbard RC, Fells G, Gadek J *et al.* (1991) Neutrophil accumulation in the lung in alpha1-antitrypsin deficiency: spontaneous release of leukotriene B4 by alveolar macrophages. *J. Clin. Invest.*;**88**:891-897.

71. Ward PA, Talamo RC. (1973) Deficiency of the chemotactic factor inactivators in human serum with alpha-1-antitrypsin deficiency. *J. Clin. Invest.*;**52**:512-519.

72. Morrison HM, Kramps JA, Afford SC *et al.* (1987) Elastase inhibitors in sputum from bronchitis patients with and without alpha1-proteinase inhibitor deficiency: partial characterization of a hitherto unquantified inhibitor of neutrophil elastase. *Clin. Sci.*;**73**:19-28.

73. Anderson R, Theron AJ, Richards GA *et al.* (1991) Passive smoking by humans sensitizes circulating neutrophils. *Am. Rev. Respir. Dis.*;**144**:570-574.

74. Takahashi H, Nukiwa T, Basset P, Crystal RG. (1988) Myelomonocytic cell lineage expression of the neutrophil elastase gene. *J. Biol. Chem.*; **263**:2543-2547.

75. MacNee W. (1997) Chronic obstructive pulmonary disease from science to the clinic: the role of glutathione in oxidant-antioxidant balance. *Monaldi Arch. Chest Dis.*;**52**:479-485.

76. Rahman I, MacNee W. (1996) Oxidant/antioxidant imbalance in smokers and in chronic obstructive pulmonary disease. *Thorax*;**51**:348-50.

77. Repine JE, Bast A, Lankhorst I and the Oxidative Stress Study Group. (1997) Oxidant stress and chronic obstructive pulmonary disease. *Am. J. Resp. Crit. Care Med.*;**156**:341-357.

78. Cantin AM, Fells GA, Hubbard RC, Crystal RG. (1990) Antioxidant macromolecules in the epithelial lining fluid of the normal human lower respiratory tract. *J. Clin. Invest.*;**86**:962-971.

79. Cooper B, Creeth JM, Donald ASR. (1985) Studies of the limited degradation of mucus glycoproteins : the mechanism of the peroxide reaction. *Biochem. J.*;**228**:615-626.

80. Cross CE, Halliwell B, Allen A. (1984) Antioxidant protection : a function of tracheobronchial and gastointestinal mucus, *Lancet*;**1**:1328-1330.

81. Hu M-L, Louie S, Cross CE, Motchnik P, Halliwell B. (1993) Antioxidant protection against hypochlorous acid in human plasma. *J. Lab. Clin. Med.*;**121**:257-262.

82. Gum JR. (1992) Mucin genes and the proteins they encode: structure diversity and regulation. *Am. J. Respir. Cell Moll. Biol.*;**7**:557-564.

83. Cantin AM, North SL, Hubbard RC, Crystal RG. (1987) Normal alveolar epithelial lung fluid contains high levels of glutathione. *J. Appl. Physiol.*;**63**:152-157

84. Linden M, Hakansson L, Ohlsson K, Sjodin K, Tegner H, Tunek A, Venge P. (1989) Glutathione in bronchoalveolar lavage fluid from smokers is related to humoral markers of inflammatory cell activity. *Inflammation*;**13**:651-658.

85. Rahman I, Li XY, Donaldson K, Harrison DJ, MacNee W. (1995) Glutathione homeostasis in alveolar epithelial cells in vitro and lung in vivo under oxidative stress. *Am. J. Physiol. : Lung Cell Moll. Biol.*;**269**:L285-L292.

86. Pacht ER, Kaseki H, Mohammed JR, Cornwell DG, Davis WR, (1988) Deficiency of vitamin E in the alveolar fluid of cigarette smokers influence on alveolar macrophage cytotoxicity. *J. Clin. Invest.*;**77**:789-796.

87. Bui MH, Sauty A, Collet F, Leuenberger P. (1992) Dietary vitamin C intake and concentrations in the body fluids and cells of male smokers and non-smokers. *J. Nutr.*;**122**:312-336.

88. McGowan SE, Parenti CM, Hoidal JR, Niewoehner DW. (1984) Differences in ascorbic acid content and accumulation by alveolar macrophages from cigarette smokers and non-smokers. *J. Lab. Clin. Med.*;**104**:127-134.

89. McCusker K, Hoidal J. (1990) Selective increase of antioxidant enzyme activity in the alveolar macrophages from cigarette smokers and smoke-exposed hamsters. *Am. Rev. Respir. Dis.*;**141**:678-682.

90. Kondo T, Tagami S, Yoshioka A, Nishumura M, Kawakami Y. (1994) Current smoking of elderly men reduces antioxidants in alveolar macrophages. *Am. J. Respir. Crit. Care Med.*;**149**:178-182.

91. York GK, Pierce TH, Schwartz LS, Cross CE. (1976) Stimulation by cigarette smoke of glutathione peroxidase system enzyme activities in rat lung. *Arch. Environ. Health*;**31**:286-290.

92. Toth KM, Berger EM, Buhler CJ, Repine JE. (1986) Erythrocytes from cigarette smokers contain more glutathione and catalase and protect endothelial cells from hydrogen peroxide better than do erythrocytes from non-smokers. *Am. Rev. Respir. Dis.*;**134**:281-284.

93. Pratico D, Basili S, Vieri M, Cordova C, Violi F, Fitzgerald FA. (1997) Chronic obstructive pulmonary disease associated with an increase in urinary levels of isoprostane $F_2\alpha$-III an index of oxidant stress. *Am. J. Resp. Crit. Care Med.*;**158**:1709-1714.

94. Rahman I, Morrison D, Donaldson K, MacNee W. (1996) Systemic oxidative stress in asthma COPD and smokers. *Am. J. Respir. Crit. Care Med.*;**154**:1055-1060.

95.   Noguera A, Busquets X, Sauleda J, Villaverde JM, MacNee W, Agusti AGN. (1999) Expression of adhesion molecules and g-proteins in circulating neutrophils in COPD. *Am. J. Respir. Crit. Care Med.*; In press

96.   Brown DM, Drost E, Donaldson K, MacNee W. (1995) Deformability and CD11/CD18 expression of sequestered neutrophils in normal and inflamed lungs. *Am. J. Respir. Cell Moll. Biol.*;**13**:531-539

97.   Duthie GG, Arthur JR, James WPT. (1991) Effects of smoking and vitamin E on blood antioxidant status. *Am. J. Clin. Nutr.*;**53**:1061S-1063S.

98.   Morrow JD, Frei B, Longmire AW, Gaziano JM. Lynch SM, Shyr Y, Strauss WE, Oates A, Roberts LJ II. (1995) Increase in circulating products of lipid peroxidation (F_2-isoprostanes) in smokers. *New Engl. J. Med.*; **332**:1198-1203.

99.   Lapenna D, Mezzetti D, Giola SD, Pierdomenico SD, Daniele F, Cuccurullo F. (1995) Plasma copper and lipid peroxidation in cigarette smokers. *Free Rad. Biol. Med.*;**19**:849-85.

100. O'Neill CA, Halliwell B, Van der Vliet A, Davis PA, Packer L. Tritschler H, Strohman WJ, Rieland T, Cross CE, Reznick AZ. (1994) Aldehyde-induced protein modifications in human plasma : Protection by glutathione and dihydrolipoic acid. *J Lab. Clin. Med.*;**124**:359-370.

101. Reznick AZ, Cross CE, Hu ML, Suzuki YJ, Khwaja S, Safadi A, Motchnik PA, Packer L, Halliwell B. (1992) Modification of plasma proteins by cigarette smoke as measured by protein carbonyls formation. *Biochem. J.*;**286**:607-611.

102. Cross CE, O'Neill CA, Reznick AZ, Hu ML, Marcocci L, Packer L, Frei B. (1993) Cigarette smoke oxidation of human plasma constitutents. *Ann. N.Y. Acad. Sci. USA.*;**686**:72-90.

103. Petruzzelli S, Hietanen E, Bartsch H, Camus AM, Mussi A, Angeletti CA, Saracci R, Giuntini C. (1990) Pulmonary lipid peroxidation in cigarette smokers and lung patients. *Chest*;**98**:930-935.

104. Bridges AB, Scott NA, Parry GJ, Belch JJF. (1993) Age, sex, cigarette smoking and indices of free radical activity in healthy humans. *Eur. J. Med.*;**2**:205-208.

105. Duthie GG, Arthur JR, James WPT. (1991) Effects of smoking and vitamin E on blood antioxidant status. *Am. J. Clin. Nutr.*;**53**: 1061S-1063S.

106. Mazzetti A, Lapenna D, Pierdomenico SD, Calafiore AM, Costantini F, Riario-Sforza G, Imbastaro T, Neri M, Cuccurullo F. (1995) Vitamins E, C and lipid peroxidation in plasma and arterial tissue of smokers and non-smokers. *Atherosclerosis.*;**112**:91-99.

107. Antwerpen LV, Theron AJ, Myer MS, Richards GA, Wolmarans L, Booysen U. (1993) Cigarette smoke-mediated oxidant stress, phagocytes, vitamin C, vitamin E and tissue injury. *Ann. N.Y. Acad. Sci. USA.*;**686**:53-65.

108. Pelletier O. (1970) Vitamin C status of cigarette smokers and non-smokers. *Am. J. Clin. Nutr.*;**23**:520-528.

109. Chow CK, Thacker R, Bridges RB, Rehm SR, Humble J, Turbek J. (1986) Lower levels of vitamin C and carotenes in plasma of cigarette smokers. *J. Am. Coll. Nutr.*;**5**:305-312.

110. Theron AJ, Richards GA, Rensburg AJ, Van der Merwe CA, Anderson R. (1990) Investigation of the role of phagocytes and antioxidant nutrients in oxidant stress mediated by cigarette smoke. *Int. J. Vitam. Nutr. Res.*;**60**:261-266.

111. Barton G, Roath OS. (1976) Leukocytic ascorbic acid in abnormal leukocyte states. *Int. J. Vitam. Nutr. Res.*;**46**:271-274.

112. Hemilla H, Roberts P, Wikstrom M. (1984) Activated polymorphonuclear leukocytes consume vitamin C. *FEBS Letts.*;**178**:25-30.

113. Bui MH, Sauty A, Collet F, Leuenberger P. (1992) Dietary vitamin C intake and concentrations in the body fluids and cells of male smokers and non-smokers. *J. Nutr.*;**122**:312-6.

114. Cross CE, O'Neill CA, Reznick AZ, Hu ML, Marcocci L, Packer L, Frei B. (1993) Cigarette smoke oxidation of human plasma constitutents. *Ann. N. Y. Acad. Sci. USA*;**686**:72-90.

115. Van der Vliet A, Smith D, O'Neill CA, Kaur H, Darley-Usmar V, Cross CE, Halliwell B. (1994) Interactions of peroxynitrite and human plasma and its constitutents : oxidative damage and antioxidant depletion. *Biochem. J.*; **303**:295-301.

116. Petruzzelli S, Puntoni R, Mimotti P, Pulera N, Baliva F, Fornai E, Giuntini C. (1997) Plasma 3-nitrotyrosine in cigarette smokers. *Am. J. Respir. Crit. Care Med.*;**156**:1902-1907.

117. Lucey EC, Stone PJ, Breuer R et al (1985) Effect of combined human neutrophil cathepsin G and elastase on induction of secretory cell metaplasia and emphysema in hamsters with in vitro observations on elastolysis by these enzymes. *Am. Rev. Respir. Dis.* **132**, 362-366.

118. Sommerhoff CP, Nadel JA, Basbaum CB, Caughey GH. (1990) Neutrophil elastase and cathepsin G stimulate secretion from cultured bovine airway gland serous cells. *J. Clin. Invest.*;**85**:682-689.

119. Adler KB, Holden-Stauffer WJ, Repine JE. (1990) Oxygen metabolites stimulate release of high molecular weight glycoconjugates by cell and organ cultures of rodent respiratory epithelium via an arachidonic acid-dependent mechanism. *J. Clin. Invest.*;**85**:75-85.

120.   Amitani R, Wilson R, Rutman A *et al.* (1991) Effects of human neutrophil elastase and *Pseudomonas aeruginosa* proteinases on human respiratory epithelium. *Am. J. Respir. Cell Moll. Biol.*;**4**:26-32.

121.   Mulier B, Rahman I, Watchorn T, Donaldson K, MacNee W, Jeffery PK. (1998) Hydrogen peroxide-induced epithelial injury: the protective role of intracellular non-protein thiols (NPSH). *Eur. Respir. J.*;**11**:384-391.

122.   Chan-Yeung M, Dy Buncio A. (1984) Leukocyte count smoking and lung function. *Am. J. Med.*;**76**:31-37.

123.   Richards GA, Theron AJ, van der Merwe CA, Anderson R. (1989) Spirometric abnormalities in young smokers correlate with increased chemiluminescence responses of activated blood phagocytes. *Am. Rev. Respir. Dis.*;**139**:181-187.

124.   Anderson R, Theron AJ, Richards GA, Myers MS, Rensburg AJV. (1991) Passive smoking by human sensitizes circulating neutrophils. *Am. Rev. Respir. Dis.*; **144**:570-574.

125.   Schunemann HJ, Muti P, Freudenheim JL, Armstrong D, Browne R, Klocke RA, Trevisan M. (1997) Oxidative stress and Lung Function. *Am. J. Epiderm.*;**146**:939-948.

126.   Britton JR, Pavord ID, Richards KA, Knox AJ, Wisniewski AF, Lewis AA, Tattersfield E, Weiss TS. (1995) Dietary antioxidant vitamin intake and lung function in the general population. *Am. J. Respir. Crit. Care Med.*;**151**:1383-1387.

127.   Sridhar MK, Galloway A, Lean MEJ, Banham SW. (1994) An out-patient nutritional supplementation programme in COPD patients. *Eur. Respir. J.*; **7**:720-724.

128.   Steinberg FM, Chait A. (1998) Antioxidant vitamin supplementation and lipid peroxidation in smokers *Am. J. Clin. Nutr.*;**68**:319-327.

129.   Jeffery PK. (1998) Structural and inflammatory changes in COPD: a comparison with asthma. *Thorax*;**53**:129-136.

130.   Keating SVM, Collins PD, Scott DM, Barnes PJ. (1996) Differences in interleukin-8 and tumour necrosis factor-induced sputum from patients with chronic obstructive pulmonary disease or asthma. *Am. J. Respir. Crit. Care Med.*;**153**:530-534.

131.   Rahman I, MacNee W. (1998) Role of transcription factors in inflammatory lung diseases. *Thorax*;**53**:601-612.

132.   Watchorn T, Mulier B, MacNee W. (1998) Does increasing intracellular glutathione inhibit cytokine-induced nitric oxide release and Nf-κB activation. *Am. J. Resp. Crit. Care Med.*;**157**:A889.

133.   Parmentier M, Drost E, Hirani N, Rahman I, Donaldson K MacNee W, Antonicelli F. Thiol antioxidants inhibit neutrophil chemotaxis by decreasing release of IL-8 from macrophages and pulmonary epithelial cells. *Am. J. Resp. Crit. Care Med.* In press

134.   Jimenez LA, Thomson J, Brown D, Rahman I, Hay RT, Donaldson K, MacNee W. PM10 particles activate NF-κB in alveolar epithelial cells. *Am. J. Resp. Crit. Care Med.* In press

135.   Li XY, Rahman I, Donaldson K, MacNee W. (1996) Mechanisms of cigarette smoke induced increased airspace permeability. *Thorax*;**51**:465-471.

136.   Rahman I, Lawson MF, Smith CAD, Harrison CJ, MacNee W. (1996) Induction of γ-glutamylcysteine synthetase by cigarette smoke is associated with AP-1 in human alveolar epithelial cells. *FEBS Letts.*;**396**:21-25.

137.   Rahman I, Bel A, Mulier B, Lawson MF, Harrison DJ, MacNee W, Smith CAD. (1996) Transcriptional regulation of γ-glutamylcysteine synthetase-heavy subunit by oxidants in human alveolar epithelial cells. *Biochem. Biophys. Res. Commun.*; **229**:832-837.

138.   Rahman I, Antonicelli F, MacNee W. Molecular mechanisms of the regulation of glutathione synthesis by tumour necrosis factor-α and dexamethasone in human alveolar epithelia cells. *J. Biol. Chem.* In press

139.   Rahman I, MacNee W. (1998) Characterisation of γ-glutamylcysteine-heavy subunit gene promoter : Critical role for AP-1. *FEBS Letts.*;**427**:129-133.

140.   Gilks CB, Price K, Wright JL, Churg A. (1998) Antioxidant gene expression in rat lung after exposure to cigarette smoke. *Am J Path*;**152**:269278.

141.   Muller T, Gebel S. (1998) The cellular stress response induced by aqueous extracts of cigarette smoke is critically dependent on the intracellular glutathione concentration. *Cardinogenesis*;**19**:797-801.

142.   Muller T. (1995) Expression of c-fos in quiescent Swiss 3T3 exposed to aqueous cigarette smoke fractions. *Can. Res.*;**55**:1927-1932.

143.   Silverman EK, Speizer FE. (1996) Risk factors for the development of chronic obstructive pulmonary disease. *Med. Clin. Nor. Am.*;**80**:501-522.

144.   Sandford AJ, Weir TD, Pare PD. (1997) Genetic risk factors for chronic obstructive pulmonary disease. *Eur Respir J*;**10**:1380-1391.

145.   Huang S-L, Su C-H, Chang S-C. (1997) Tumor necrosis factor-α gene polymorphism in chronic bronchitis. *Am. J. Respir. Crit. Care Med.*;**156**:1436-1439.

146. Smith CAD, Harrison DJ. (1997) Association between polymorphism in gene for microsomal epoxide hydrolase and susceptibility to emphysema *Lancet*;**350**:630-633.

147. Clausen J. (1991) The influence of antioxidants on the enhanced respiratory burst reaction in smokers. *Annal. N. Y. Acad. Sci. USA*;**629**:337-341.

148. Davis WB, Pacht ER, Spatafora M, Marin WJ II. (1998) Enhanced cytotoxic potential of alveolar macrophages from cigarette smokers. *J. Lab. Clin. Med.*;**111**:293-298.

149. Hoshino E, Shariff R, Van Gossum A et al (1990) Vitamin E suppresses increased lipid peroxidation in cigarette smokers. *J. Parenter. Enter. Nutr.*; **40**:300-305.

150. Pacht ER, Kaseki H, Mohammed JR, Cornwell DG, Davis WR. (1988) Deficiency of vitamin E in the alveolar fluid of cigarette smokers Influence on alveolar macrophage cytotoxicity. *J. Clin. Invest.*;**77**:789-796.

151. MacNee W, Bridgeman MME, Marsden M, Drost E, Lannan S, Selby C, Donaldson K. (1991) The effects of N-acetylcysteine and glutathione on smoke-induced changes in lung phagocytes and epithelial cells. *Am. J. Med.*; **90**:60s-66s.

152. Ross D, Norbeck K Moldeus P. (1985) The generation and subsequent fate of gluthionyl radicals in biological systems. *J. Biol. Chem.*; **260**:15028-15032.

153. Marrades RM, Roca J, Barbera J. Jover L de, MacNee W, Rodriguez-Roisin R. (1997) Nebulized glutathione induces bronchoconstriction in patients with mild asthma. *Am. J. Respir. Crit. Care. Med.*;**156**:425-430.

154. Meister A, Anderson ME. (1983) Glutathione. *Ann. Rev. Biochem.*;**52**:711-760.

155. Karlsen RL, Grofova I, Malthe-Soren D, Cross CE, C A O'Neill A Z Reznick M L Hu L Marcocci L Packer and B Frei (1993) Cigarette smoke oxidation of human plasma constitutents. *Ann. N. Y. Acad. Sci. USA*;**686**:72-90.

156. Bridgeman MME, Marsden M, MacNee W, Flenley DC, Ryle AO. (1991) Cysteine and glutathione concentrations in plasma and bronchoalveolar lavage fluid after treatment with N-acetylcysteine. *Thorax*;**46**:39-42.

157. Bridgemen MME, Marsden M, Selby C, Morrison D, MacNee W. (1994) Effect of N-acetyl cysteine on the concentrations of thiols in plasma bronchoalveolar lavage fluid and lining tissue. *Thorax*;**49**:670-675.

158. Bowman G, Backer U, Larsson S, Melander B, Wahlander L. (1983) Oral acetylcysteine reduces exacerbation rate in chronic bronchitis. *Eur. J. Respir. Dis.*;**64**:405-415.

159. Rasmusse JB, Glennow C. (1988) Reduction in days of illness after long-term treatment with N-acetylcysteine controlled-release tablets in patients with chronic bronchitis. *Eur. J. Respir. Dis.*;**1**:351-355.

160. British Thoracic Society Research Committee. (1985) Oral N-acetylcysteine and exacerbation rates in patients with chronic bronchitis and severe airways obstruction. *Thorax*;**40**:823-835

161. Gillissen A, Jaworska M, Orth M, Coffiner M, Maes P, App EM, Cantin AM, Schultze-Werninghaus G. (1997) Nacystelyn a novel lysine salt of N-acetylcysteine to augment cellular antioxidant defence in vitro. *Respir. Med.*;**91**:159-168.

162. Nagy AM, Vanderbist F, Parij N, Maes P, Fondu P, Neve J. (1997) Effect of the mucoactive drug Nacystelyn on the respiratory burst of human blood polymorphonuclear neutrophils. *Pulm. Pharmacol. Ther.*; **10**:287-292.

163. Anderson ME, Powrie F, Puri R, Meister A. (1985) Glutathione monoethyl ester : preparation uptake by tissues and conversion to glutathione. *Arch. Biochem. Biophys.*;**239**:538-548

164. Tsan M, White JE, Rosano CL. (1989) Modulation of endothelial GSH concentrations : effect of exogenous GSH and GSH monoethyl ester. *J. Appl. Physiol.*;**66**:1029-1034.

165. Tsan MF, Phillips PG. L-2-oxothiazolidine-4-carboxylate protects cultured endothelial cells against hyperoxia-induced injury. *Inflammation* **12**:113-121.

Acute Lung Injury: From Inflammation to Repair
G.J. Bellingan and G.J. Laurent (Eds.)
IOS Press, 2000

The Neutrophil in Acute and Chronic Lung Disease

Robert A. Stockley

Department of Medicine
Queen Elizabeth Hospital, Birmingham, UK

1   Introduction.

The polymorphonuclear leukocyte is the most abundant of all circulating leukocytes (5×10^{11}). It has a key role in the secondary defence of the lung and in health only small numbers can be found within the airways. However, once the local defences have been overwhelmed by the inhalation of foreign material, including bacteria, the neutrophil becomes the major "fast response" cell moving in large numbers to sites of inflammation and infection. Once in the lung the neutrophils perform primary phagocytic roles, ingesting foreign material, leading to antigen digestion and bacterial killing. In order to achieve this primary function the neutrophils have a sophisticated system of cellular protein and enzymes which enable them to respond specifically, moving to the areas of infection. The importance of this cell and its sophisticated characteristics are highlighted by the recurrence and severity of infections caused by specific genetic defects of the neutrophil (see later).

2   Neutrophil kinetics.

Neutrophils are derived from the bone marrow from a pleuripotent stem cell, which produces cells of the granulocyte lineage. The neutrophil is characterised by the presence of a multi-lobed nucleus and the characteristic granules. Differentiation of the neutrophils takes place entirely within the bone marrow and several distinct stages can be recognised (Figure 1). In the first stage which takes some 5-7 days the cell differentiates from a myeloblast through the promyelocyte stage to form the myelocyte. During this phase the cell undergoes cell division and at the same time produces the primary or azurophil granules and their contents. These granules contain many of the key proteins utilised in host defence, including the proteinases elastase, proteinase 3 and Cathepsin G, antibacterial proteins such as the defensins, lysozyme and azurocidin and the enzyme myeloperoxidase used in the generation of superoxide radicals.

As the cell approaches the metamyelocyte state the secondary or specific granules and their contents are formed and the primary and secondary granules are divided up amongst the daughter cells. However, from the metamyelocyte stage onwards the cell no longer undergoes division, but matures through a recognised band cell stage to form the mature neutrophil. This whole process takes approximately 2 weeks in total and the mature cells remain in the bone marrow for approximately a further 2 days before being released into the blood where they have a short circulating half life of approximately 8 hours.

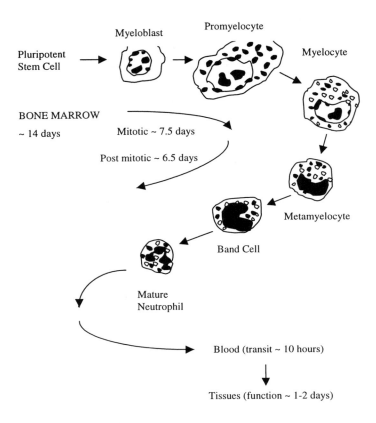

Figure 1. Diagrammatic representation of neutrophil differentiation that takes place within the bone marrow.

At any one time approximately half of the neutrophils in the circulation are believed to be "marginated", mainly within the pulmonary circulation. These cells and cells late in differentiation stored within the bone marrow can be rapidly mobilised at the onset of infection, leading to appropriate local accumulation, and sometimes the release of slightly immature (hypersegmented) cells, often referred to as a "left shift".

3   Neutrophil recruitment to the lungs.

In the presence of inflammation all neutrophils found within lung tissues are derived directly from the blood, since mature cells are no longer capable of division. Once in the tissues the cells do not recirculate and, having performed their function of phagocytosis and bacterial killing, the cells are cleared by a combination of the mucociliary escalator and the process of programmed cell death, or apoptosis. Following this latter process the cells are ingested by the macrophages as a mechanism which prevents the release of potentially tissue damaging proteinases as the cell disintegrates [1].

The process of cell recruitment consists of a series of complex events involving specific signals from the lung which activate the cells. In broad terms this involves 3 stages: cell tethering cell triggering and adhesion, and finally neutrophil migration.

4   Tethering.

Under the normal sheer stresses associated with blood flow, cells move along the edges of the vessel lumen, making contact with endothelial cells. In smaller vessels the neutrophil has to deform to pass through leading to all round cell/cell contact. As the cells move they are tethered to the endothelial cells by surface receptors called selectins. This family of adhesion molecules bind to sialyated carbohydrate groups on their counter receptors and are therefore "lectin-like" receptors. The neutrophils express L-selectin constitutively on the cell surface and the counter receptors are expressed on the endothelial cells (E-selectin and P-selectin). The P-selectin molecules are stored within the endothelial cells and translocate rapidly to the plasma membrane under the influence of inflammatory mediators [2]. In contrast E-selectin is not pre-stored but is synthesised rapidly and transported to the plasma membrane in response to inflammatory cytokines, including TNF-α, Interleukin-1β and Interleukin-8 [3].

Although this initial tethering is a weak form of attachment the importance of selectin mediated tethering is demonstrated by leukocyte adhesion deficiency II (LAD-II). This is characterised by a failure to express sialyl Lewis X, a counter receptor for E-selectin and P-selectin. Because of this deficiency neutrophils fail to migrate to inflammatory foci, resulting in recurrent bacterial infections [4].

As indicated above, selectin mediated attachment is weak and the bonds are easily broken under the influence of sheer stress forces. Because these initial adhesion events are transitory, cells can be seen to roll hesitatingly along the endothelial surface of larger blood vessels. Thus the second step in cell recruitment requires permanent strong adhesion and cell triggering.

5   Triggering and strong adhesion.

Weak tethering and rolling of the neutrophils brings them into close contact with endothelial cells. When this occurs at regions of inflammation the neutrophil will also be exposed to factors that trigger or activate other neutrophil receptors, the integrins, which are responsible for strong adhesion. The integrins are a family of transmembrane glycoproteins that are heterodimeric, consisting of 1 alpha and 1 beta sub-unit which are bound covalently. Subfamilies share common beta sub-units and the different family members have distinct alpha sub-units. With respect to the neutrophil the most important integrin is Mac-1 (CD11b-CD18). In addition LFA1 (CD11a-CD18) is also expressed but is probably less important for strong binding. Again the importance of the beta-2 integrins is illustrated by the inherited condition, LAD-1, which is due to reduced or absent expression of the beta-2 integrins, again resulting in recurrent infections [5].

The beta-2 integrins bind to intercellular counter-receptors, expressed on the endothelial cell. Mac-I binds to ICAM-I and LFA1 binds to ICAM-1, ICAM-2 and ICAM-3. Again the expression of integrins and ICAM-1 is modulated by a variety of pro-inflammatory factors. For instance, integrin adhesiveness is increased on neutrophils by factors such as Interleukin-8, as well as those derived from micro-organisms such as N-formyl-methionyl-leucyl-phenylalanine.

Although the beta-2 integrins can be mobilised and expressed on the cell surface following activation of the neutrophil, the majority of the initial triggering is the direct result of conformational change in a proportion of the integrin molecule, inducing a greater affinity for the counter receptors [6]. On the other hand. whereas ICAM-2 appears to be constitutively expressed by endothelial cells, ICAM-1 expression can be increased [7] Again several cytokines can influence this process and ICAM-1 expression is increased by

Interleukin-1, TNF-α as well as bacterial lipopolysaccharide. Thus several of the same factors released from an inflammatory focus can lead to activation of neutrophil integrins as well as up-regulation of their counter-receptors on endothelial cells. This whole process results in strong binding of the neutrophil at the site of inflammation.

6   Neutrophil migration.

Neutrophils migrate in response to many chemotactic factors. These would include lnterleukin-8, C5a, LTB4 and bacterial peptides. Again the neutrophil constitutively expresses the appropriate receptors on the cell surface and receptor binding by the appropriate chemoattractant leads to polarisation of the cell and movement of receptors towards the point of polarisation. At this stage the cell moves in the direction of increasing concentrations of a chemoattractant. As the concentration of the chemoattractant increases the cell moves more rapidly until the concentration exceeds a certain optimal value. whereupon the cell becomes greatly activated and starts to move at random. With reference to the formyl peptide, FMLP, this differential response of chemotaxis and activation can be seen to be optimal at concentrations that 2 orders of magnitude different (Figure 2).

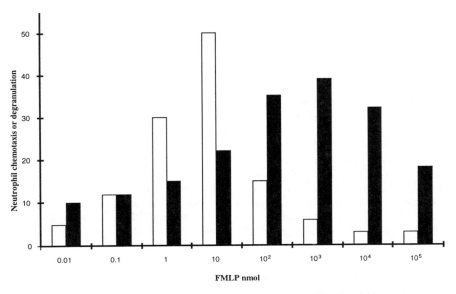

Figure 2. The individual responses of neutrophils to FMLP are shown. The closed histogram represents concentration dependent chemotactic response whereas the open histograms represent the degranulation response. The y axis is "Neutrophil chemotxis or degranulation".

In addition to being able to move and become activated by different concentrations of the same chemoattractant, the neutrophil can also move differentially when exposed to different chemoattractants. For instance when the cell has moved effectively along the primary gradient to a saturating non-orientating concentration of an initial attractant, it can subsequently move effectively to a secondary distant agent [81. This whole process may be of importance in the lung, for instance by enabling the cell to move into the airway in response to a natural chemoattractant made by the lung (Interleukin-8) and then subsequently in the airway to move towards bacteria that are releasing bacterial peptides, such as FMLP. This whole concept of cell adhesion and migration is indicated in Figure 3.

BIDIRECTIONAL MIGRATION

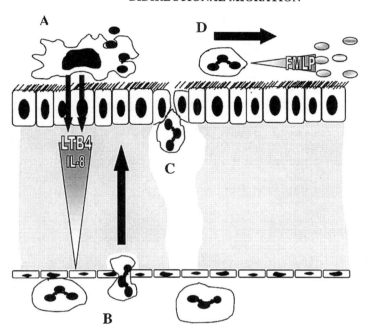

Figure 3. The influence of different chemotactic factors on neutrophil recruitment into the airway. A: Macrophage phagocytosis of bacteria leads to activation of the cell and release of chemoattractants such as LTB4 and 1L-8. B: Receptor binding of the chemoattractants lead to polarisation of the neutrophil and movement from the vascular space into the lung. C: Migration through the extracellular matrix leads to destruction of connective tissue as the cell continues to move up the chemoattractant gradient to its source within the airway. D: Having arrived at the source of release of the initial chemoattractants the neutrophil may now change direction, moving towards a different chemoattractant such as FMLP or other bacterial products being released within the airway.

The process of cell migration involves several steps. Firstly, the cell has to move from the strong binding between the beta-2 integrins and the ICAMs. This process probably involves proteolytic cleavage of ICAM. Although the enzymes responsible for this have yet to be clearly identified. recent data has indicated that as the neutrophil becomes activated release of neutrophil elastase at the site of adhesion will cleave ICAM-1[9]. At this point the neutrophil will move between endothelial cells, again involving a cleavage process by separating the strong adhesion between cells due to cadherins. As the neutrophil moves through the basement membrane beneath the endothelial cells it enters the area where long-lived connective tissue is present. This tight matrix would restrict the movement of a large cell, such as the neutrophil. However once again it is likely that release of proteolytic enzymes facilitate this process [10]. As the connective tissue is digested the cell moves to the epithelial cell layer and hence into the airways. The implication of this digestive process as the cell moves will be covered in more detail later.

7   Neutrophil effector functions.

Several of the factors which lead to neutrophil activation and migration are also responsible for activating the cell effector functions responsible for killing and elimination of micro-organisms. The mechanisms employed by the neutrophil include phagocytosis, the respiratory burst and the release of cytotoxic peptides and proteins.

8   Phagocytosis.

Ingestion of bacteria by the phagocytic process is a prelude to intracellular killing. Although the neutrophil can ingest bacterial particles this process is made much more efficient by the process of opsonisation whereby immunoglobulin binds to surface bacterial antigens. This process leads to the activation of complement and both the immunoglobulin heavy chain and the complement factor, C3, will then bind to specific receptors on the surface of the neutrophil. Ingested bacteria are then trapped and encapsulated within the phagolysosome where they are killed and degraded. The killing is achieved by both the respiratory, burst and the action of cytotoxic proteins.

9   The respiratory burst.

The neutrophil respiratory burst results in the release of oxidative products. originating from the membrane-bound NADPH oxidase system. Again the importance of this mechanism is illustrated by chronic granulomatous disease in which recurrent infections occur because the phagocytic cells of the affected individuals are unable to generate the products of the respiratory burst [11]. The superoxide production starts with the reduction of oxygen by NADPH to form the superoxide radical (O_2). These radicals can react spontaneously (dismute) to produce molecular oxygen and hydrogen peroxide but this reaction is also catalysed by superoxide dismutase. The reduction of hydrogen peroxide to water, or to hyperchlorous acid in the presence of chloride is catalysed by the enzyme myeloperoxidase which is present in the azurophil granules. They and others are incredibly toxic and have a very short range of activity. These products are released in high concentrations into the phagolysosome where they destroy the ingested bacteria.

10   Cytotoxic proteins.

The granules of the neutrophil contain a variety of proteins with a cytotoxic potential. Most of these are located within the azurophil granules and include the defensins (the family of 4 cyclic single chain peptides with a molecular weight of about 4,000) they include a human neutrophil peptides (HNP) 1-3 and are highly toxic to fungi and enveloped viruses as well as bacteria. Azurocidin is very similar in structure to the proteinases, elastase and cathepsin G and again has a major cytotoxic activity. The proteinases are found both within the primary azurophil granules as well as the specific granules. However the class of proteinase differs between the two granules. The serine proteinases are present within the primary granules whereas the metalloproteinases are largely confined to the specific granules.

The three most important serine proteinases in the primary granules are elastase cathepsin G and proteinase 3. Although these enzymes may have more important roles neutrophil elastase [12] and also cathepsin G [13] have been shown to be bactericidal.

although the bactericidal activity of cathepsin G is not dependent upon its enzyme activity. Again the importance of these proteinases is demonstrated by a genetic deficiency, the Chediak-Higashi syndrome. This is associated with the development of abnormal granules which (in the mature cell) contains none of the serine proteinases in the azurophil granule. The neutrophils have normal phagocytic activity and respiratory burst but are deficient in bacterial killing, leading to recurrent pulmonary infections [14].

11   The neutrophil in lung damage.

Although the neutrophil is clearly an important cell in host defence, interest in recent years has concentrated on the ability of the cell to cause "bystander" damage to the lung, resulting in the generation of both acute and chronic lung disease. The neutrophil products of respiratory burst have the ability to damage normal bronchial cells, resulting in cell death [15] and may play an important role in the severe destruction seen in the acute respiratory distress syndrome [16]. In addition the proteinases released by the neutrophil have been shown to cause many effects, both *in vitro* and *in vivo* within the lung that are typical of the pathological changes seen in patients with chronic lung disease. The role of these enzymes and in particular the serine proteinase neutrophil elastase, has been the topic of extensive research over the last 20-30 years. The studies date from the observation in 1963 of the development of severe emphysema in young individuals who were found to have a deficiency of the serine proteinase α-l-antitrypsin [17]. Because the association was so strong it was felt that α-l-antitrypsin in some way protected the lungs from the development of emphysema. At the same time animal experiments had shown that a proteolytically enzyme (papain) had the ability to produce emphysematous-like lesions in the lungs of experimental animals [18]. It therefore seemed reasonable to assume that an enzyme normally inhibited by α-l-antitrypsin was responsible for the development of emphysema in the deficient subjects.

Over the next few years animal experimentation indeed showed that enzymes. particularly with the ability to digest lung elastin could produce lesions in experimental animals that were typical of the emphysematous changes seen in human disease. Eventually neutrophil elastase was isolated and shown to produce emphysema in experimental animals [19]. This resulted in the closing of the loop and it was believed that release of neutrophil elastase by neutrophils recruited to the lungs of individuals with α-l-antitrypsin deficiency resulted in excessive degradation of lung elastin leading to the development of disease. This concept led to the now well accepted proteinase/antiproteinase theory of the development of emphysema.

However few subjects who developed emphysema had clearly demonstrable deficiency of α-l-antitrypsin. Studies were therefore undertaken to determine mechanisms that could lead to a functional deficiency of α-l-antitrypsin, creating the same proteinase/antiproteinase balance that was seen in true deficient subjects. Of importance were studies that demonstrated that cigarette smoke (a major risk factor in the development of emphysema) and oxidants released from activated neutrophils could inactivate the α-l-antitrypsin by oxidation of the active site methionine [20]. It therefore seemed a logical step to assume that in a cigarette smoker inactivation of α-l-antitrypsin led to a secondary deficiency which resulted in the development of emphysema. The major problem with this whole concept, however, is the fact that the majority of people who smoke do not develop significant emphysema, so a simple biochemical explanation would not appear to be appropriate [21].

In recent years, however, the process of connective tissue degradation by neutrophils migrating into the lung has been studied in more detail. This has led to the understanding of connective tissue degradation and more particularly why α-l-antitrypsin deficiency renders the individual more susceptible to the development of more severe disease at a younger age.

12   Cell migration.

As indicated previously the migration of the neutrophil through the close knit interstitial tissues requires degradation to create a pathway and to facilitate cell movement. Early studies by Campbell and colleagues [22] suggested that, as the neutrophil bound tightly to connective tissue, its activation resulted in digestion of the matrix proteins connective tissue, even in the presence of proteinase inhibitors. This process did not require oxidation of the α-l-antitrypsin since it also occurred when using neutrophils from subjects with chronic granulomatous disease (where the neutrophil respiratory burst is deficient). Initially it was thought that the tight adherence between the neutrophil and the connective tissue matrix did not allow free diffusion of the inhibitor into the subcellular space, thereby effectively excluding it and facilitating tissue degradation by local release of proteinases. However, more recently, studies by Liou and Campbell, both on theoretical [23] and practical grounds [24], have demonstrated that the process represents a true proteinase/ antiproteinase imbalance. These studies demonstrated that the concentration of neutrophil elastase within the single azurophil granule was of the order of 5 mMolar. As the cell is activated the azurophil granules move to the surface of the cell and are extruded [25]. At this point the enzyme diffuses away from the granule and as it does so its concentration gradually decreases. When the concentration falls almost 2 orders of magnitude to the physiological concentration of the surrounding proteinase inhibitors, the activity of the enzyme becomes totally inactivated. This process is known as quantum proteolysis. The mechanism clearly results in a supra-physiological concentration of an enzyme at the surface of the activated neutrophil resulting in an obligate area of proteolytic destruction of connective tissue near the cell, creating a pathway. As the cell moves and the enzyme diffuses further away from the granule, it will eventually be inactivated by the surrounding inhibitors, thereby limiting the area of damage. However, the relationship between the concentration of enzyme and the distance moved away from the cell is exponential. This means that once the concentration of the surrounding inhibitor falls below 10 μMolar the area of damage produced by release of enzyme from a single granule becomes excessively large. Subjects with α-l-antitrypsin deficiency have plasma concentrations of α-l-antitrypsin which is approximately 5 μMolar and therefore below the threshold of 10 μMolar which is necessary to tightly control the area of connective tissue digestion.

This observation therefore explains why subjects with α-l-antitrypsin deficiency are particularly susceptible to connective tissue destruction by migrating neutrophils. However this process also enables us to understand how connective tissue destruction leading to emphysema can also occur in subjects who have normal concentrations of α-l-antitrypsin. Clearly the migration of a single neutrophil leads to connective tissue destruction. Lung elastin is a long-lived connective tissue in health [26]. Once it is destroyed, although it may re-accumulate [27], it does so in an amorphous fashion that disrupts the delicate architecture of the lung. Thus the more neutrophils that move into the lung and the longer the period of time over which they do so, the more likely is the subject to develop significant connective tissue destruction and therefore (potentially) emphysematous change. Thus it is not necessary to implicate proteinase inhibitor deficiency in the generation of emphysema, but merely to implicate neutrophils, their activation and recruitment.

With this concept in mind it is possible to construct a putative pathway that results in the generation of emphysema by neutrophils.

13   Emphysema.

Emphysema is predominantly a condition of smokers. However it is clear that the majority of smokers do not develop clinically significant emphysema and it is only a susceptible minority (approximately 15%) that do so. There have, however been very few studies that have investigated the possibility that neutrophil recruitment might explain this susceptibility. The majority of studies that have been carried out to investigate the pathogenic processes involved in emphysema have compared the lung inflammation in healthy smokers with that in healthy non smokers. Clearly with only a susceptible minority it is likely that group data from healthy smokers will largely overwhelm the susceptibility factor expressed only by a small proportion of them. In addition studies in patients who already have established emphysema are difficult to interpret since the presence of the disease itself may alter the results. However with these problems in mind there clearly are studies within the literature that indicate the potential mechanisms involved.

McCrea and colleagues [28] studied lung lavages from healthy smokers and non smokers. They identified that a small proportion of subjects who smoked had high concentrations of Interleukin-8 in their peripheral lung secretions. In addition the secretions from these 2 subjects showed increased neutrophil chemotactic activity. Interleukin-8 is one of the major lung chemoattractants for the neutrophil [29]. Thus it would be expected that in the individuals who smoked who had high concentrations of interleukin-8 would recruit a greater number of neutrophils, leading to an increased neutrophil burden. This process over many years would lead to accumulation of a greater degree of connective tissue damage in this subset of individuals. Clearly, however, although this process seems sensible to explain the development of disease, long term studies will be necessary to confirm its importance.

Nevertheless studies are continuing into the role of Interleukin-8. For instance cigarette smoking itself leads to the production of Interleukin-8 by bronchi al epithelial cells [30]. It is therefore possible that in certain individuals the regulation of Interleukin-8 by epithelial cells may be abnormal, either because of a genetic defect or a secondary effect, perhaps related to latent virus infections [31].

14   Studies in subjects with emphysema.

There have been very few studies of factors that can influence proteolytic degradation of the lung in subjects with emphysema. However in 1987 Burnett and colleagues [32] demonstrated that neutrophils from subjects with established emphysema behaved in an abnormal way. Firstly the cells showed an enhanced chemotactic response to a standard chemoattractant compared to cells from healthy smoking matched individuals and subjects with another inflammatory lung disease (bronchiectasis). The implications of this study was that the release of normal amounts of chemoattractants from the lungs would result in greater neutrophil recruitment and hence an increase in proteolytic destruction as the cells migrate.

In addition to this difference in neutrophil function the authors also observed that the capacity of the neutrophils to damage connective tissue was also increased. This was not because the cells had been already activated since the addition of a further activating agent led to an even greater increase in the proteolytic destructive capability of these cells [32]. Both of these neutrophil responses were shown to be related to an increase in the number of chemotactic peptide receptors on the surface of the cell [33]. The overall implications from these studies was were: (a) an increase in the number of neutrophil be recruited to the lungs in response to a standard chemoattractant; (b) the cells themselves would have a greater destructive potential as they migrated. However, as indicated previously, the interpretation of these data is hampered by the fact that the presence of disease itself may influence the results. However, more recently, further information has provided potential supporting data.

Although it is well recognised that cigarette smoking in susceptible individuals leads to the development of emphysema it is equally well recognised that cessation of smoking leads to a reduction in the destructive process and thus progression of emphysema. Thus in the study of emphysematous subjects. Identification of the pathogenic process requires the study of patients with a similar degree of lung disease who either continue to smoke or who have ceased smoking. Cessation of smoking should lead to a reduction in the putative pathogenic factor. With this in mind there has been a lot of interest recently in the role of other proteinases in the development of emphysema. For instance studies have shown that collagenase activity, in lung lavage from patients with emphysema is increased [34]. Nevertheless when the data was divided into current smokers and ex smokers, the concentration of collagenase was similar. On the other hand the concentrations of neutrophil elastase showed a clear difference with the values being higher in current smokers and much lower in subjects who ceased smoking, thus implicating neutrophil elastase as a major potential pathogenic factor, supporting previous concepts as well as many *in vitro* and *in vivo* studies. With this in mind our own group has studied the concentration of the chemoattractant peptide, interleukin-8, in the lung secretions from emphysematous smokers and ex smokers. The data shows a significant reduction in interleukin-8 concentrations in subjects who had ceased to smoke (Figure 4). The net result of a reduction in Interleukin-8 would be a concomitant reduction in neutrophil migration and hence neutrophil mediated interstitial damage resulting in a reduction of disease progression.

In summary, there is much supporting data from *in vitro* and *in vivo* experiments, both in experimental animals and man to implicate many factors involved in neutrophil recruitment and connective tissue destruction by neutrophils, via the release of neutrophil elastase leading to the development of emphysema. At this stage it is unlikely that further insights in to the process will be obtained until intervention studies with specific elastase inhibitors have taken place.

15   The role of neutrophil in chronic bronchial disease.

Although bronchial disease has received much less attention than emphysema there is increasing information that implicates the neutrophil in the development and perpetuation of the condition. Biopsies from patients with chronic bronchial disease demonstrate that the neutrophil is often present [35]. Indeed neutrophils are regularly identified in the airway secretions from patients with chronic bronchial disease. In the sputum from patients with COPD the numbers are often low, whereas in other conditions such as bronchiectasis with and without cystic fibrosis neutrophil numbers are excessive.

In COPD in the stable clinical state the airway secretions contain low but detectable concentrations of neutrophil elastase [36]. However in most of these samples the activity of the enzyme is undetectable, largely because it is overwhelmed by the concentrations of inhibitors such as α-1-antitrypsin and secretory leukoprotease inhibitor in the secretions. However during acute exacerbations of COPD, due to bacterial infection the concentration of neutrophil elastase is vastly increased and its activity, is easily detectable [36] as it overwhelms the concentrations of the local inhibitors. A similar situation is often present in patients with bronchiectasis, even in the stable clinical state and may represent an excessive neutrophil response to bacterial colonisation (see later).

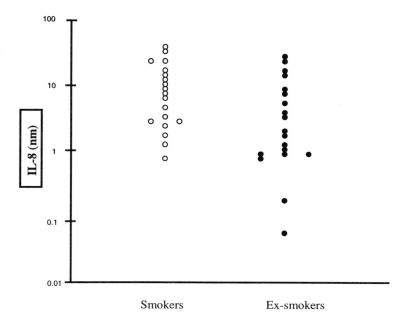

Figure 4. Sputum concentrations of Interleukin-8 in subjects with COPD matched for age and sex. Each point represents the result from the sputum of an individual patient. The groups are divided into current smokers and ex-smokers.

Neutrophil elastase has been shown to have a major effect on the airways. *In vitro* inflammation and airways damage can be shown in experimental animal models within a short period of instilling neutrophil elastase [37]. In addition, with time, experimental animals, developed mucus gland hyperplasia [38] and the addition of neutrophil elastase to mucus glands results in excessive mucus secretion [39]. Neutrophil elastase added to ciliated epithelium results in a significant slowing of the beat frequency of the cilia [40] and in addition neutrophil elastase has been shown to damage immunoglobulins [41] and the important opsonophagocytic receptor, C3bi [42], resulting in major impairment of critical host defences of the lung. These features are recognised in patients with bronchial disease. where epithelial damage may be present and patients often complain of mucus production with a cough resulting in expectoration of sputum. In addition studies have shown that mucociliary clearance is reduced [43] and the impairment of these important host defences result in bacterial colonisation [44]. This latter process may in fact become self-perpetuating (see later).

The processes involved are poorly understood. As indicated at the start of this chapter the neutrophil is an important cell in host defence. Its primary function is to move to areas of infection to facilitate removal of the invading organism. With this in mind the process of initiation, amplification and resolution of the inflammatory process will be key elements in the response to infection.

16   Initiation.

Bacterial are continually inhaled into the airway, although in health these are usually cleared by the normal mucociliary escalator, or the resident airway macrophages. When the bacterial load exceeds the ability of these primary defences, either due to defence impairment or the inhalation of large numbers of bacteria, the secondary defences are activated. The exact mechanisms for initiation of the process are poorly understood. However as indicated previously it will result from activation of the neutrophil and endothelial adhesion molecules as well as the generation of an appropriate chemoattractant gradient. Endotoxin from bacteria has been shown to stimulate epithelial cells to release the pro-inflammatory cytokines TNF-α and IL-1β [45]. which increase ICAM-I expression on endothelial cells [7]. Endotoxin and TNF-α also cause epithelial cells to produce interleukin-8 which will form a chemoattractant gradient for the neutrophil from the epithelial cells through to the endothelium. In addition the resident alveolar macrophage will release both Interleukin-8 and LTB4 during the process of bacterial phagocytosis adding to the chemoattractant gradient.

17   Amplification.

As neutrophils move into the airway they degrade connective tissue releasing peptides that may be chemoattractant in their own right. Similarly the activation of the neutrophils results in further release of the chemoattractants, LTB4 and interleukin-8. that will also add to the chemoattractant gradient. Finally as the neutrophils release elastase this can activate complement factor 5, resulting in the release of C5a [46] which is also chemoattractant and it has been suggested that leukocyte elastase may also activate epithelial cells to release even more interleukin-8 [47]. The release of neutrophil elastase in the airway would normally be inhibited by secretory leukoproteinase inhibitor. However studies have shown that active elastase reduces epithelial cell release of this inhibitor [48] and this process may facilitate elastase activity in the airway. Although this process may be detrimental it is possible that this plays a significant role in host defences, since elastase itself has been shown to be bactericidal [12] and perhaps, more importantly, elastase results in mucus release from mucus glands [39] that will entrap the bacteria, leading to their clearance by expectoration.

18   Resolution.

The recruitment of the neutrophil to the airway leads to an increase in bacterial phagocytosis. If sufficient this will sterilise the airway, leading to a reduction of the pro-inflammatory cytokine release due to the presence of bacteria. In addition the neutrophils will become less activated. resulting in a reduction of their release of chemoattractants and elastase. The inactivation of elastase is further facilitated by the development of inflammation. Elastase has been shown to increase protein leakage between epithelial cells [49] and this together with the acute phase response will result in recruitment of large quantities of α-l-antitrypsin from the circulation into the airway. The net effect will be to increase the ability of the airway secretions to inhibit neutrophil elastase, thereby negating its potentially harmful effects and the beneficial ones that should no longer be needed.

19   Perpetuation.

Although the above process may be self-limiting and short-lived, as for instance in the development of acute bronchial infection or pneumonia, there may be instances in which the process becomes self-perpetuating.

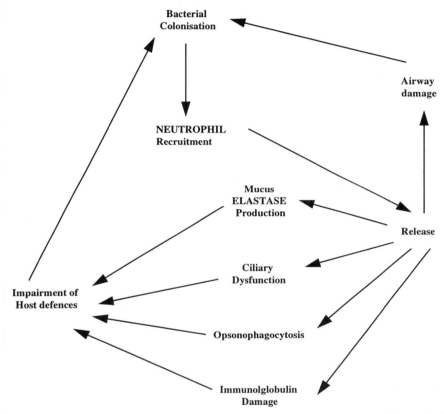

Figure 5. Diagrammatic representation of perpetuation of the inflammatory response in subjects with airway damage. Persistent bacterial colonisation leads to continual neutrophil recruitment. On activation the neutrophil releases many products including neutrophil elastase which in its own right leads to further airway damage facilitating bacterial colonisation. In addition elastase release results in excess mucus production, ciliary dysfunction a reduction in the opsonophagocytic potential of the cells and damage to immunoglobulins. These in turn lead to further major impairment of host defences, facilitating further bacterial colonisation.

Significant irreversible impairment of lung defences due to airway damage may result in colonisation of the airways by bacteria. If the numbers of organisms present are high the ensuing inflammatory process may be insufficient to sterilise the airway resulting in a perpetuation of the process and the destructive side effects. Such a situation is thought to be the case in patients with bronchiectasis and cystic fibrosis, resulting in a vicious circle of inflammation (Figure 5).

The central role of bacteria in this process is clearly indicated by studies of empirical treatment of antibiotic therapy in patients with bronchiectasis who have a high degree of neutrophil influx. Within a short period of time of commencement of antibiotic therapy neutrophil influx (as indicated by myeloperoxidase concentration) is dramatically reduced. The free elastase activity within the airway secretions becomes undetectable and protein leakage from lung inflammation is also reduced [50]. These changes are associated with a reduction in chemoattractant concentrations of interleukin-8 and LTB4 [51]. However in patients with bronchiectasis with and without cystic fibrosis the response to antibiotic therapy is often short-lived. This is probably related to failure to completely sterilise the airway but in addition reflects the major impairment of host defences relate to the excessive bronchial damage.

Whatever the underlying cause the process reverses rapidly (often within days) and the lung returns to its inflamed state [50]. Occasionally long term antibiotic treatment of such patients is indicated to ensure continued reduction of the inflammatory process and in some cessation of therapy after several months is not always associated with a return to the inflamed state.

Clearly such studies in the airways are complex and difficult to dissect. The importance of various mediators can only be hypothesised until specific intervention studies are available. If neutrophils play a key role in the development and perpetuation of bronchial disease the processes involved remain yet to be clarified. Severe bronchial damage can occur in patients with acute pneumonia and the development of bronchiectasis has been described in subjects with a variety of acute lung infections [52]. Nevertheless most patients who develop such infections do not go on to develop extensive bronchial damage. Furthermore some patients colonised by bacteria have minimal or low grade inflammatory responses and whether these are the cause of the neutrophil recruitment resulting in epithelial damage and mucus gland hyperplasia rather than the other way round remains to be determined.

In summary the neutrophil is a critical cell involved in defence of the lung. It is highly designed for a fast response when required and has a major destructive armamentarium to facilitate sterilisation of the airway. However the processes of cell recruitment and activation also have the potential to cause pathological and destructive changes within the airway. The development of these changes may result in major impairments in host defence that give rise to long-lived and progressive sequelae. The features that determine whether resolution or progression occurs remain to be clarified.

References.

1.   Meagher, L., J. Savill, A. Baker, R. Fuller and C. Haslett. (1992) Phagocytosis of apoptotic neutrophils does not induce macrophage release of thromboxane B2. *J. Leuk. Biol.* **52:** 269-273.

2.   Bonfanti, R., B. Furie, B. Furie, D. Wagner. (1989) PADGEM (GMP 140) is a component of the weibel-PALADE bodies of human endothelial cells. *Blood* **73:**109-1112.

3.   Pevilacqua, M., J. Pober, D. Mendrick, R. Cotran, M. Gimbrone. (1987) Identification of an inducible endothelial-leukocyte adhesion molecule. *Proc. Natl. Acad. Sci* **84:** 9238-9242.

4.   Etzioni, A., M. Frydman S. Pollack *et al.* (1992) Brief report: recurrence of ear infections caused by a novel leukocyte adhesion deficiency *New Engl. J Med.* **327:**1789-1792.

5.   Anderson D., T. Springer. (1987) Leukocyte adhesion deficiency: an inherited defect of the Mac-1, LFA-1 and p150,95 glycoproteins. *Ann. Rev. Med.* **38:**175-194.

6.   Carbano, C. and N. Hogg. (1993) Ligand intercellular adhesion molecule 1 has a necessary role in activation of integrin lymphocyte function - associated molecule *Proc. Natl. Acad. Sci. USA* **90:**5838-5842.

7.   Pober, J., M. Gimbrone, L. Lapierre *et al.* (1986) Overlapping patterns of activation of human endothelial cells by Interleukin-1, tumour necrosis factor and immune interferon. *J Immunol.* **137:** 1893-1896.

8.   Campbell JJ, Foxman EF, Butcher EC (1997) Chemoattractant receptor cross talk as a regulatory mechanism in leukocyte adhesion and migration. *Eur J Immunol* **27:** 2571-8

9.   Champagne B, Tremblay P, Cantin A, St Pierre Y (1998) Proteolytic cleavage of ICAM-1 by human neutrophil elastase. *J Immunol* **161:** 6398-405

10. Okada S, Kita H, George TJ, Gleich GJ, Leiferman KM (1997) Migration of eosinophils through basement membrane components in vitro: role of matrix metalloproteinase-9. *Am. J. Respir. Cell Moll. Biol.* **17:** 519-28

11. Curnutte JT, Whitten DM, Babior BM (1974) Defective superoxide production by granulocytes from patients with chronic granulomatous disease. *N. Engl. J. Med.* **290:** 593-7

12. Belaaouaj A, McCarthy R, Baumann M, Gao Z, Ley TJ, Abraham SN, Shapiro SD (1998) Mice lacking neutrophil elastase reveal impaired host defence against gram negative bacterial sepsis. *Nat Med* **4:** 615-8

13. Odeberg H, Olsson I (1976) Mechanisms for the microbicidal activity of cationic proteins of human granulocytes. *Infect Immun* **14:** 1269-75

14. Blume RS, Wolff SM (1972) The Chediak-Higashi syndrome: studies in four patients and a review of the literature. *Medicine (Baltimore)* **51:** 247-80

15. Weiss S. J., J. Young, A. F. LoBugho, A. Slivka N. F. Nimeh. (1981) Role of hydrogen peroxide in neutrophil-mediated destruction of cultured endothelial cells. J. *Clin. Invest.* **68:** 714-721.

16. Ward, P. A., G. 0. Till, R. Kunkel, C. Beachamp. (1983) Evidence for the role of hydroxyl radical in complement and neutrophil dependent tissue injury. *J Clin. Invest:* **72:** 789-801.

17. Laurell, C-B., S. Eriksson. (1963) Electrophoretic alpha-I-globulin pattern of serum in alpha-1-antitrypsin deficiency. *Scand. J. Clin. Lab. Invest.* **15:** 132-140.

18. Gross. P., E. A. Pfitzer. E. Tolker, M. A. Babiak, M. Kaschak. (1965) Experimental emphysema. Its production with papain in normal and silicotic rats. *Arch. Environ. Health.* **11:** 50-58.

19. Senior, R. M., H. Tegner, C. Kuhn, K. Ohlsson. B. C. Starcher, J. A. Pierce. (1977) Induction of pulmonary emphysema with human leukocyte elastase. Ann. *Rev. Respir. Dis.* **116:** 469-475.

20. Johnson. D.. J. Travis. (1979) The oxidative inactivation of human alpha-I -proteinase inhibitor. Further evidence for methionine at the reactive centre. *J. Biol. Chem.* **254:** 4022-4026.

21. Stockley, R. A. 1987. Alpha-1-antitrypsin and the pathogenesis of emphysema. *Lung.* **165:** 61-77.

22. Campbell, E. J., R. M. Senior, J. A. MacDonald, D. L. Cox. (1982) Proteolysis by neutrophils. Relative importance of cell-substrate contact and oxidative inactivation of proteinase inhibitors in vitro. *J Clin. Invest.* **70:** 845-852.

23. Liou, T. G., E. J. Campbell. (1995) Non-isotropic enzyme-inhibitor interactions: a novel non-oxidative mechanism for quantum proteolysis by human neutrophils. *Biochemistry;* **34:** 16171-16177.

24. Liou T. G., F. J. Campbell. (1996) Quantum proteolysis resulting from release of single granules by neutrophils: a novel non-oxidative mechanism of extracellular proteolytic activity. *J. Immunol.* **157:** 2624-2631

25. Owen C. A., M. A. Campbell, P. L. Sannes S. S. Bonkedes. E. J. Campbell. (1995) Cell-surface-bound elastase in Cathepsin G in human neutrophils. A novel non-oxidative mechanism by which neutrophils focus and preserve catalytic activity of serine proteinases. *J. Cell Bio.* **131:** 775-789.

26. Shapiro, S., D. J. A. Pierce. S. K. Endicott and E. J. Campbell. (1991) Marked longevity of human lung parenchymal elastic fibres deduced from prevalence of D-aspartate and nuclear weapons - related radiocarbon. *J. Clin Invest.* **87:** 1828-1834.

27. Kuhn, C., J. Slodkowska, T. Smith, B. Starcher. (1980) The tissue response to exogenous elastase. *Bull. Europ. Physiopath. Respir.* **16** (suppl): 127-13.

28. McCrea, K. A., J. E. Ensor, K. Nall. E. R. Blicker and J. D. Hasday. (1994) Altered cytokine regulation in the lungs of cigarette smokers. *Am. J Respir. Crit. Care Med.* **150:** 696-703.

29. Richman-Eisenstat, J. B. Y., P. G. Jorens, C. A. Hibert, I. Ueki and J. A. Nadel. (1993) Interleukin-8: an important chemoattractant in sputum of patients with chronic inflammatory airway diseases. *Am. J. Physiol;* **264:** L413-L418.

30. Tadashi, M.. D. J. Vomberger, A. B. Thompson, R. A. Robbins, A. Heires and S. Rennard. (1997) Cigarette smoking induces Interleukin-8 release from human bronchial epithelial cells. *Am. J Respir. Crit. Care Med.* **155:** 1770-1776.

31. Vitalis, T. Z., I. Kern, A. Croome, H. Behzad, S. Hayashi. J. C. Hogg. (1998) The effect of latent adenovirus 5 infection on cigarette smoke-induced lung inflammation. *Eur. Respir. J.* **11:** 664-669.

32. Burnett D., A. Chamba. S. L. Hill, R. Stockley. (1987) Neutrophils from subjects with chronic obstructive lung disease show enhanced chemotaxis and extracellular proteolysis. *Lancet,* **ii:** 1043-1046.

33. Stockley, R. A., R. A. Grant, C.G. Llewellyn-Jones, S. L. Hill and D. Burnett. (1994) Neutrophil Formyl Peptide Receptors: relationship to peptide induced responses and emphysema. *Am. J. Respir. Crit. Care Med.* **149:** 464-468.

34. Finlay. C. A., K. J. Russell. K. J. McMahon. E. M. D'Arcy. J. B. Masterston. M. X. Fitzgerald, C. M. O'Connor. (1997) Elevated levels of matrix metalloproteinases in bronchoalveolar lavage fluid on emphysematous patients. *Thorax.* **52:** 502-506.

35.   Di Stefano, A.. P. Maestrelli. A. Roggeri. G. Turato, S. Calabro. A. Potena. C. F. Mapp, A. Ciaccia, L. Covalev, L. NI. Fabbri *et al.* (1994) Up-regulation of adhesion molecules in the bronchial mucosa of subjects with chronic obstruction bronchitis. *Am. J. Respir Crit. Care Med:* **141:** 803-810.

36.   Stockley, R. A. and D. Burnett. (1979) Alpha1-antitrypsin and leukocyte elastase in infected and non-infected sputum. *Am. Rev. Respir. Dis.* **120:** 1081-1086.

37.   Suzuki, T., W. Wang, J-T. Linn, K. Sherato, H. Mitsuhashi and H. Inoue. (1996) Aerosolised human neutrophil elastase induces airways constriction and hyper-responsiveness with protection by intravenous pre-treatment with half-length secretory leukoprotease inhibitor. *Am. J. Respir. Crit. Care Med.* **153:** 1405-1411.

38.   Lucey, E. C., P. J. Stone, R. Breuer, P. C. Christensen. J. D. Calore, A. Catanese. C. Franz-Blau and G. L. Snider. (1985) Effect of combined human neutrophil Cathepsin G and elastase on induction of secretory cell metaplasia and emphysema in hamsters with in vitro observations on elastolysis by these enzymes. *Am. Rev. Respir. Dis.* **132:** 362-366.

39.   Sommerhoff: C. P.. J. A. Nadel. C. B. Basbaum and G. H. Caughey. (1990) Neutrophil elastase and Cathepsin G stimulate secretion from cultured bovine airway glands serous cells. *J. Clin. Invest.* **85:** 682-689.

40.   Smallman, L. A., S. L. Hill. R. A. Stockley. (1984) Reduction of ciliary beat frequency in vitro by sputum from patients with bronchiectasis: a serine proteinase effect. *Thorax* **39:** 663-667.

41.   Solomon, A. (1978) Possible role of PMN proteinases in immunoglobulin degradation and amyloid formation. In: K. Havemaun A. Janoff. editors. Neutrophil Proteinases of Human Polymorphonuclear Leukocytes. Urban and Schwarzenberg. Baltimore: pp 423-438.

42.   Berger M., R. U. Sorensen, M. F. Tosi, D. G. Dearborn, G. Doring. (1989) Complement receptor expression on neutrophils at an inflammatory site, the *Pseudomonas* infected lung in cystic fibrosis. *J. Clin. Invest.* **84:** 1302-1313.

43.   Currie, D. C., D. Pavia, J. F. Agnew *et al.* (1987) Impaired tracheo-bronchial clearance in bronchiectasis. *Thorax* **42:** 126-130.

44.   Monso. E., J. Ruiz, A. Rosell, J. Manterola, J. Fiz. J. Morera and V. Ausina. (1995) Bacterial infection in chronic obstruction pulmonary disease. A study of stable and exacerbated outpatients using the protected specimen brush. *Am. J. Respir. Crit. Care Med.* **152:** 1316-1320.

45.   Khair, 0. A., J. F. Devalia, M. M. Abdilaziz, R. J. Sapsford and R. J. Davis. (1994) Effect of Haemophilus influenzae endotoxin on synthesis of IL-6, IL-8, TNF-α. and expression of ICAM-1 in cultured human bronchial epithelial cells. *Eur. Respir. J.* **7:** 2109-2116.

46.   Venger. P. and I. Olsson. (1975) Cationic proteins of human granulocytes. VI. Effects on the complement system and mediation of chemotactic activity. *J. Immunol:* **115:** 1505-1508.

47.   Nakamura, H.. K. Yoshimura, N. G. McElvania and R. G. Crystal. (1994) Neutrophil elastase in respiratory epithelial lining fluid of individuals with cystic fibrosis induces interleukin-8 gene expression in a human bronchial epithelial cell line. *J. Clin. Invest* **89:** 1478-1484.

48.   Sallenave, J., M. J. Schulman, J. Crossley. M. Jordana and J. K. Gauldie. (1994) Regulation of secretory leukocyte proteinase inhibitor (SLPI) and elastase specific inhibitor (ESI-elafin) in human airway epithelial cells by cytokines and neutrophilic enzymes. *Am. J. Respir. Cell Moll. Biol.* **11:** 733-741.

49.   Petersen, M. W., M. E. Walter and S. D. Nygaard. (1995) Effect of neutrophil mediators on epithelial permeability. *Am. J. Respir. Cell Moll. Biol.* **13:** 719-727.

50.   Stockley, R. A,. S. L. Hill and H. M. Morrison. (1984) Effect of antibiotic treatment on sputum in bronchiectatic outpatients in a stable clinical state. *Thorax.* **39:** 414-419.

51.   Mikami, M., C. G. Llewellyn-Jones, D. Bayley, S. L. Hill, R. Stockley. (1998) Chemotactic activity of sputum from patients with bronchiectasis. *Am. J. Respir. Crit. Care Med.* **157:** 723-728

52.   Stockley R. A. (1996) Bronchiectasis. In: Oxford Textbook of Medicine (3rd. ed). Eds. D. J. Weatherall. J. G. G. Ledingham. D. A. Warrall. Oxford Univ. Press. Oxford. Pp. 2755-2766.

Acute Lung Injury: From Inflammation to Repair
G.J. Bellingan and G.J. Laurent (Eds.)
IOS Press, 2000

Reducing Inflammation by the Induction of Tolerance

Gerard F. Hoyne

Respiratory Medicine Unit, University of Edinburgh Medical School, Teviot Place,

Edinburgh EH8 9AG, UK

Abstract: CD4+ T cells play an important role in allergic sensitisation and thus represent a key target for allergen immunotherapy. In this report we describe how mucosal administration of a single allergen derived peptide of the house dust mite allergen Der p 1, which contains the immunodominant T cell epitope, can render mice profoundly unresponsive to an immuogenic challenge with the intact protein. The development of tolerance is associated with the induction of regulatory CD4+ T cells which can transfer tolerance and mediate linked suppression. We have been investigating how CD4+ T cells are selected for a regulatory function *in vivo* and have identified a role for the evolutionary conserved Notch signalling pathway in this process. These studies provide a new insight into the regulation of T cell growth in the peripheral circulation and have important implications in the development of new therapeutic strategies.

1   Introduction.

The goal of specific immunotherapy is to immunize with allergens or their derivatives so as to reduce the severity of clinical disease in patients without compromising their ability to develop immunity to other pathogens. It is established that allergen sensitization in genetically susceptible individuals arises as a result of an inappropriate immune responses to environmental allergens and is characterized by increased production of allergen-specific immunoglobulin E (IgE) [1]. The allergic response is accompanied by the infiltration of inflammatory cells such as mast cells, basophils and eosinophils, into the airways which release histamine, leukotrienes and other inflammatory mediators [2]. This heterogeneity in the cell types and mediators contributing to allergic inflammation provides several potential targets in immunotherapy.

2   House dust mite allergy.

Allergens derived from the *Dermatophagoides spp.* of house dust mite (HDM) are a significant cause of allergic disease in humans, and exposure to HDM in early childhood represents a significant risk factor for the development of allergic disease in later life [3]. There is increasing evidence to suggest that allergen-specific CD4+ T helper (Th) cells play an important role in allergic sensitization, through the nature of the cytokines they secrete when activated [4]. CD4+ Th cells from atopic patients display a Th2 phenotype and predominantly secrete cytokines such as IL-4, IL-5 and IL-13 which are central in the regulation of allergic inflammatory responses and these cells are an obvious target of specific immunotherapy [5-9]. CD4+ T cells are activated following the recognition of peptide fragments of allergen occupying the antigen combining site of MHC class II molecules [4,10]. Therefore, considerable interest has been generated in the use of allergen derived T cell epitopes, presented to the immune system in the form of peptides, to inhibit the functional activity of specific Th2 cells or to promote the induction of Th1 cells, which appear to dominate the response to allergens in non-atopic individuals [5,8,9,11]. Furthermore there is evidence to suggest that *in vivo* the T cell repertoire of atopic individuals contains a population of long lived allergen reactive CD4+ T cell clones [12]. A recent study by Wedderburn and colleagues showed that these clones shared the same T cell receptor genes suggesting they recognize a restricted number of epitopes, and are maintained *in vivo* by chronic exposure to environmental allergens [12]. Underlying the importance of CD4+ Th cells in the allergic response, it has been shown that successful desensitization to grass pollen allergens correlated with a decease in Th cell function but without a reduction in the levels of specific IgE patients [13-16]. Therefore immunotherapy based on altering the qualitative and/or quantitative nature of the cellular immune response may be beneficial. Improvements in the treatment of HDM allergy in the future may therefore rely on our ability to specifically target allergen-specific CD4+ T cells to inhibit their function *in vivo*. Using a murine model we have studied the ability of immuogenic peptides derived from the major HDM allergen, Der p 1, to induce antigen-specific tolerance *in vivo*.

3   The mucosal delivery of antigen.

The mucosal delivery of antigen can lead to systemic priming but invariably, the outcome of the immune response is the development of long lasting peripheral tolerance [17,18]. We have demonstrated that intranasal administration of the immunodominant T cell epitope (residues 110-131) of the group 1 allergen of *D. pteronyssinus*, Der p 1, at high doses induces profound and long lasting tolerance [19,20]. The peptide which is specific for CD4+ Th cells when given under tolerogenic conditions induces a transient activation of T cells prior to the development of tolerance [19]. We have shown that the induction of tolerance does not require CD8+ T cells and is not associated with a shift in cytokine production by CD4+ T cells [19,21]. A feature of mucosal tolerance generated by intranasal administration of peptide is the phenomenon of linked suppression, whereby tolerance induced to a single epitope leads to inhibition of responses to all CD4+ epitopes in Der p 1, provided that the tolerant mice were challenged with the intact protein [19-22] . Furthermore, we have demonstrated that this phenomenon is mediated by regulatory CD4+ T cells [23].

Linked suppression (or bystander suppression) has also been demonstrated for experimental models of peripheral tolerance involving self and transplantation antigens [24-32]. In each of these cases linked suppression is mediated by regulatory CD4+ T cells. The processing and presentation of multiple epitopes originating within the same protein (Der p 1) by a single or neighbouring antigen presenting cell (APC) is thought to bring regulatory and naive T cells into close proximity and this would facilitate the transfer of inhibitory signals between the T cells [23]. It has been proposed that the release of immunosuppressive cytokines, such as IL-10, IL-4 and TGF-β1, provide the negative signals that mediate the inhibitory effects observed in linked suppression [11, 16, 18]. However, we have been unable to detect either TGF-β or Th2-type cytokine production by T cells from tolerant mice when restimulated with peptide *in vitro* [5, 23]. Therefore, it is possible that the mechanism of linked suppression in this system requires direct cell contact between the regulatory and naive T cells, similar to that which has been reported for bystander suppression mediated by anergic human T cell clones *in vitro* [33,34].

4   The *Notch* receptor.

During development cell-cell interactions are critical in enabling equivalent precursor cells to adopt alternate cell fates. One signalling pathway that has the capacity to regulate such cell fate decisions in various tissues, and in a diverse range of organisms, is that controlled by the *Notch* receptor [35,36]. *Notch* is an evolutionary conserved transmembrane protein that was first described as a neurogenic gene in *Drosophila* since mutations in the *Notch* gene affected whether precursor cells differentiated as either neurones or epidermal cells [37]. In *Caenorhabditis elegans* vulva precursor cells can give rise to two distinct cell lineages known as the ventral uterine (VU) cell, a primary fate, or the anchor (AC) cell a secondary cell fate [38,39]. The choice between these lineages is regulated by a cell contact dependent process involving signalling through the Notch receptor *Lin-12* and the ligand *Lag-2* [40]. The choice between the neuronal versus epidermal cell lineages or between AC and VU is believed to arise from random fluctuations in expression of the *Notch* receptor and its ligand(s) during early development [35,40]. *Notch* signalling is induced when one precursor cell expresses high levels of the ligand and neighbouring (receiving) cells express high levels of *Notch*.

Vertebrate *Notch* homologues have now been identified in various tissues and it is anticipated that they will play a role not only in embryogenesis, but also in the regulation of cell growth and differentiation of adult tissues [41 and references therein]. *Notch* can bind to two separate ligands, Delta and Serrate [37] of which there are vertebrate homologues and the receptor and its ligands are co-expressed within the same tissues [42-46]. In the immune system, cell fate decisions occur within the thymus, where T cell precursors choose between the TCRαβ and TCRγδ lineages, and then again when TCRαβ cells differentiate into CD4+ and CD8+ single positive cells [47,48]. Recent studies by Robey and colleagues suggest that Notch signalling is required at both of these stages of T cell development [49,50]. However, at present, little is known of the physiological function of the Notch ligands in mediating these cell fate decisions of thymocytes. *Notch* signalling also appears to play a very important role in the regulation of haematopoiesis [51-54]. Moreover, recent studies suggest that *Notch* signalling is sensitive to the presence of cytokines and this may influence the differentiation of precursor cells [51].

One of the best studied roles for *Notch* signalling is its function in neurogenesis in *Drosophila* and in the AC/VU decision in *C. elegans* where it functions in a process known as lateral signalling [13,15,17,36,40]. This involves a cell contact dependent mechanism whereby the Notch receptor on one precursor cell binds to its ligand (Delta or Lag-2 in flies and worms respectively) on a neighbouring cells, and this can influence whether a precursor follows one of two fates, a neural or epidermal fate in the case of the fly or the AC or VU fate in worms [13,36,40]. This prompted us to investigate if Notch/Delta interactions between T cells might contribute to peripheral tolerance and mediate linked suppression through an analogous process of lateral signalling.

4.1   *Delta1*.

We have found that *Notch1* and *Notch 2* are expressed in peripheral lymphoid tissues of mice and that they also co-express on a limited number of cells the ligands *Delta1* and *Serrate1*. We find that *Delta1* is expressed by T cells and that there is a marked increase in the number of *Delta1* expressing cells in draining lymph nodes following the intranasal administration of high dose peptide as determined by *in situ* hybridisation. The expression of *Delta1* was maximal 4 days after peptide treatment and had declined by day 8, whereas *Delta1* transcripts in unprimed mice were barely detectable. Rechallenging tolerant mice with an immunogenic dose of Der p 1 in adjuvant resulted in the *Delta1* expression at levels higher than those observed following tolerance induction. In contrast, increased expression of *Delta1* was not seen following the active immunisation of non-tolerant mice with Der p 1 in adjuvant. These results demonstrate that *Delta1* expression is transiently upregulated as a consequence of peptide-induced tolerance. Furthermore, *Delta1* is re-expressed when tolerant mice are exposed to antigen rechallenge under conditions that normally prime and, therefore, this suggests that *Notch/Delta1* signalling may be important in the maintenance as well as in the induction of peripheral tolerance.

4.2   *Notch/Delta1* signalling.

In order to investigate the function of *Notch/Delta1* signalling in T cell tolerance we have used retroviral gene mediated transfer to overexpress the murine *Delta1* gene in p 1, 110-131 specific CD4+ T cells. We have injected irradiated *Delta1*+ or control infected T cells into naive mice and immunised them with Der p 1 or ovalbumin (OVA) in adjuvant to examine what influence the Delta1 expression might have on the ability of mice to generate a response to the HDM allergen. Our results have shown that lymph node T cells from the mice that had received the *Delta1*+ T cells failed to proliferate when rechallenged with Der p 1 *in vitro* but this inhibitory effect was not observed if mice were immunized with an irrelevant antigen, OVA. These studies were extended and responses to minor (e.g.. residues 81-102) as well as the dominant T cell epitope in Der p 1 were examined. We observed that the adoptive transfer of the *Delta1*+ T cells, reactive with p 1, 110-131, inhibited responses to both the dominant and minor determinants. The results of these experiments suggest that CD4+ T cells expressing *Delta1* mediate similar effects to regulatory T cells selected by high dose of peptide in that they induce antigen specific peripheral T cell tolerance and mediate linked suppression.

The induction of nasal tolerance is associated with a transient activation and expansion of CD4+ T cells [19] which eventually gives rise to a population of antigen-specific regulatory T cells. Although it remains unclear how T cells are selected for a regulatory role *in vivo*, we have begun to focus on a potential mechanism to explain how these cells can mediate linked suppression in tolerance. Our results suggest that in peripheral tolerance induced by nasally administered peptide, *Delta1* is transiently expressed on the surface of T cells destined to become regulatory cells and this can ligate *Notch*, which is constitutively expressed on naive T cells. Following immunization of tolerant mice with intact protein, APCs in the environment of the draining lymph node will be able to present multiple epitopes of the antigen on its surface. This would provide the opportunity for regulatory and naive T cells to cluster at the membrane of the same APC, presenting both the major and minor T cell epitopes. Recognition of antigen by the regulatory T cells would lead to increased surface expression of the *Delta1* ligand and this could ligate *Notch* on the surface of the neighbouring naive T cell. The outcome of *Notch-Delta* signalling in this instance is to prevent the clonal expansion and differentiation of the naive T cell, and thus mediate linked suppression.

A feature of lateral signalling in neurogenesis is that *Notch-Delta* signalling does not lead to cell death, on the contrary, cells receiving the *Notch* signal are kept alive but are prevented from growing and differentiating. Thus, because of its fundamental role in the development of various tissues, the *Notch* signalling pathway may have been utilised by the immune system in order to regulate the growth and differentiation of cells. Consistent with this idea is the emerging role for Notch signalling in the regulation of haematopoietic progenitors [24, 19, 23, 29, 51-55] . Further studies shall hopefully shed light on how the expression of the ligand *Delta1* is controlled following T cell receptor signalling.

Acknowledgements.

This work was supported by the Medical Research Council and a Sir Henry Wellcome Commemorative Award for Innovative Research.

References.

1. O'Hehir R. E., Hoyne, G. F., Thomas, W. R., and Lamb, J. R. (1993). House dust mite allergy. From epitopes to immunotherapy. *Eur. J. Clin. Invest.* **23**, 763-772.
2. Ishizaka A, Hasegawa N, Sakamaki F, Tasaka S, Nakamura H, Kishikawa K, Yamada A, Obata T, Sayama K, Urano T, et al (1994) Effects of ONO-1078, a peptide leukotriene antagonist, on endotoxin-induced acute lung injury. *Am J Respir Crit Care Med* **150**: 1325-31
3. Platts-Mills T. A., and Chapman, M. D. (1987). Dust mites: immunology, allergic disease, and environmental control. *J. Allergy Clin. Immunol.* **80**, 755-775.
4. O'Hehir R. E., Garman, R. D., Greenstein, J. L., and Lamb, J. R. (1991). The specificity and regulation of T-cell responsiveness to allergens. *Ann. Rev. Immunol.* **9**, 67-95.
5. Parronchi P., Macchia, D., Piccini, M.-P., Biswas, P., Simonelli, C., Maggi, E., Ricci, M., Ansari, A., and Romagnani, S. (1991). Allergen and bacterial antigen specific T cell clones established from atopic donors show a different production profile of cytokine production. *Proc. Natl. Acad. Sci. USA* **88**, 4538.
6. Punnonen J., and de Vries, J. E. (1994). IL-13 induces proliferation , Ig isotype switching and Ig synthesis in immature human foetal B cells. *J. Immunol.* **152**, 1094.
7. Varney V. A., Hamid, Q. A., Gaga, M., Ying, S., Jacobson, M., Frew, A. J., Kay, A. B., and Durham, S. R. (1993). Influence of grass pollen immunotherapy on cellular infiltration and cytokine mRNA expression during allergen induced late phase cutaneous responses. *J. Clin. Invest.* **92**, 644.
8. Wierenga E. A., Snoek, M., DeGroot, C., Chretien, I., Bos, J. D., Jansen, H. M., and Kaspenburg, M. L. (1990). Evidence for compartmentilization of functional subsets of $CD4^+$ T lymphocytes in atopic patients. *J. Immunol.* **144**, 4651-4656.
9. Yssel H., Johnson, K. E., Schneider, P. V., Wideman, J., Terr, A., Kastelein, R., and De Vries, J. E. (1992). T cell activation inducing epitopes of the house dust mite allergen *Der p* 1: Proliferation ad lymphokine production patterns by *Der p* 1 specific CD4+ T cell clones. *J. Immunol.* In press.
10. Babbitt B. P., Matsueda, G., Haber, E., Unanue, E. R., and Allen, P. M. (1986). Antigenic competition at the level of peptide-Ia binding. *Proc. Natl. Acad. Sci. U S A* **83**, 4509-4513.
11. O'Hehir R. E., Bal, V., Quint, D., Moqbel, R., Kay, A. B., Zanders, E. D., and Lamb, J. R. (1989). An *in vitro* model of allergen-dependent IgE synthesis by human B lymphocytes: comparison of the response of an atopic and a non-atopic individual to *Dermatophagoides* spp. (house dust mite). *Immunology* **66**, 499-504.
12. Wedderburn L. R., O'Hehir, R. E., Hewitt, C. R. A., Lamb, J. R., and Owen, M. J. (1993). *In vivo* clonal dominance and limited T cell receptor usage in human CD4+ T cell recognition of house dust mite allergens. Proc. Natl. Acad. Sci. USA **90**, 8214.
13. Akdis C. A., Akdis, M., Blesken, T., Wymann, D., Alkan, S. S., Müller, U., and Blaser, K. (1996). Epitope-specific T cell tolerance to phospholipase A_2 in bee venom immunotherapy and recovery by IL-2 and IL-15 *in vitro*. *J Clin Invest* **98**, 1676-1683.
14. Jutel M. P., Pichler, W. J., Skrbic, D., Uryler, A., Dahinden, C., and Muller, U. R. (1995). Bee venom immunotherapy results in a decrease of IL-4 and IL-5 and an increase in IFN-g secretion in specific allergen stimulated cultures. *J. Immunol.* **154**, 4187-4194.
15. Muller U., Fricker, M., Caraballido, J., and Blaser, K. (1995). Successful immunotherapy with T-cell epitopes of bee venom phospholipase A2 in two patients with bee venom allergy. In: New trends in allergy. Eds. J. Ring and H. Berendt. (Hamburg).
16. Secrist H., Chelen, C. J., Wen, Y., Marshall, J. D., and Umetsu, D. T. (1993). Allergen immunotherapy decreases interleukin 4 production in CD4+ T cells from allergic individuals. *J. Exp. Med.* **178**, 2123-2130.

17.   Mowat A. M. (1987). The regulation of immune responses to dietary antigens. *Immunology Today* **8**, 93-98.

18.   Weiner H. L., Friedman, A., Miller, A., Khoury, S. J., Al-Sabbagh, A., Santos, L., Sayegh, M., Nussenblatt, R. B., Trentham, D. E., and Hafler, D. A. (1994). Oral Tolerance: immunologic mechanisms and treatment of animal and human organ-specific autoimmune diseases by oral administration of autoantigens. *Ann. Rev. Immunol.* **12**, 809-837.

19.   Hoyne G. F., Askonas, B. A., Hetzel, C., Thomas, W. R., and Lamb, J. R. (1996). Regulation of house dust mite responses by inhaled peptide: transient activation precedes the development of tolerance in vivo. *Int. Immunol.* **8**, 335-342.

20.   Hoyne G. F., O'Hehir, R. E., Wraith, D. C., Thomas, W. R., and Lamb, J. R. (1993). Inhibition of T cell and antibody responses to house dust mite allergen by inhalation of the dominant T cell epitope in naive and sensitised mice. *J. Exp. Med.* **178**, 1783-1788.

21.   Hoyne G. F., Jarnicki, A. G., Thomas, W. R., and Lamb, J. R. (1997). Characterization of the specificity and duration of T cell tolerance to nasally administered peptides: A role for intramolecular epitope suppression. *Int. Immunol.* **9**, 1163-1175.

22.   Hoyne G. F., Callow, M. G., Kuo, M.-C., and Thomas, W. R. (1994). Inhibition of T cell responses by feeding peptides containing major and cryptic epitopes. Studies with the *Der p* I allergen. *Immunology* **83**, 190-195.

23.   Hoyne G. F., and Lamb, J. R. (1997). Regulation of mucosal tolerance. *Immunol. Cell Biol.* **75** : 197-201.

24.   Anderton S. M., and Wraith, D. C. (1998). Hierarchy in the ability of T cell epitopes to induce peripheral tolerance to antigens from myelin. *Eur. J. Immunol.* **28**, 1251-1261.

25.   Chen Y., Kuchroo, V. K., Inobe, J.-i., Hafler, D. A., and Weiner, H. L. (1994). Regulatory T cell clones induced by oral tolerance: suppression of autoimmune encephalomyelitis. *Science* **265**, 1237-1240.

26.   Davies J. D., Leong, L. Y. W., Mellor, A., Cobbold, S. P., and Waldmann, H. (1996). T cell suppression in transplantation tolerance through linked recognition. *J. Immunol.* **156**, 3602-3607.

27.   Le Dourain N., Corbel, C., Bandeira, A., Thomas-Vaslin, V., Modigliani, Y., Coutinho, A., and Salaun, J. (1996). Evidence for a thymus-dependent form of tolerance that is not based on elimination or anergy. *Immunol. Rev.* **149**, 35-53.

28.   Metzler B., and Wraith, D. C. (1993). Inhibition of experimental autoimmune encephalomyelitis by inhalation but not oral administration of the encephalitogenic peptide: influence of MHC binding affinity. *Int. Immunol.* **5**, 1159-1165.

29.   Qin S. X., Cobbold, S. P., Pope, H., Elliot, J., Kioussis, D., Davies, J., and Waldmann, H. (1993). "Infectious" Transplantation Tolerance. *Science* **259**, 974-977.

30.   Saoudi A., Seddon, B., Fowell, D., and Mason, D. (1996). The thymus contains a high frequency of cells that prevent autoimmune diabetes on transfer into prediabetic recipients. *J. Exp. Med.* **184**, 2393-2398.

31.   Staines N. A., Harper, N., Ward, F. J., Malmstrom, V., Holmdahl, R., and Bansal, S. (1996). Mucosal tolerance and suppression of collagen-induced arthritis (CIA) induced by nasal inhalation of synthetic peptide 184-198 of bovine type II collagen (CII) expressing a dominant T cell epitope. *Clin. Exp. Immunol.* **103**, 368-375.

32.   Wong W., Morris, P. J., and Wood, K. J. (1997). Pretransplant administration of a single donor class I major histocompatibility complex molecule is sufficient for the indefinite survival of fully allogeneic cardiac allografts. *Transplantation* **63**, 1490-1494.

33.   Lamb J. R., Skidmore, B. J., Green, N., Chiller, J. M., and Feldmann, M. (1983). Induction of tolerance in influenza virus-immune T lymphocyte clones with synthetic peptides of influenza hemagglutinin. *J. Exp. Med.* **157**, 1434-1447.

34.   Lombardi G., Sidhu, S., Batchelor, R., and Lechler, R. (1994). Anergic T cells as suppressor cells in vitro. *Science* **264**, 1587-1589.

35.   Artavanis-Tsakonas S., Matsuno, K., and Fortini, M. (1995). Notch signalling. *Science* **268**, 225-232.

36.   Simpson P. (1997). Notch signalling in development: on equivalence groups and asymmetric developmental potential. *Curr. Opin. Genet. Dev.* **7**, 537-542.

37.   Fleming R. J., Purcell, K., and Artavanis-Tsakonas, S. (1997). The NOTCH receptor and its ligands. *Trends Cell Biol.* **7**, 437-441.

38.   Seydoux G., and Greenwald, I. (1989). Cell autonomy of lin-12 function in a cell fate decision in C. elegans. *Cell* **57**, 1237-1245.

39.   Wilkinson H. A., Fitzgerald, K., and Greenwald, I. (1994). Reciprocal changes in expression of the receptor lin-12 and its ligand lag-2 prior to commitment in a C. elegans cell fate decision. *Cell* **79**, 1187-1198.

40.   Greenwald I. (1998). LIN-12/Notch signalling: lessons from worms and flies. *Genes & Dev.* **12**, 1751-1762.

41.   Robey E. (1997). Notch in vertebrates. *Curr. Opin. Genet. Dev.* **7**, 551-557.
42.   Chitnis A. B. (1995). The role of Notch in lateral inhibition and cell fate specification. *Moll. Cell. Neurosci.* **6**, 311-321.
43.   Henrique D., Adam, J., Myat, A., Chitnis, A., Lewis, J., and Ish-Horowicz, D. (1995). Expression of a *Delta* homologue in prospective neurones in the chick. *Nature* **375**, 787-790.
44.   Hrabe de Angelis M., McIntyre, J., and Gossler, A. (1997). Maintenance of somite borders in mice requires the *Delta* homologue *Dll1*. *Nature* **386**, 717-721.
45.   Laufer E., Dahn, R., Orozco, O. E., Yeo, C.-Y., Pisenti, J., Henrique, D., Abbott, U. K., Fallon, J. F., and Tabin, C. (1997). Expression of Radical fringe in limb-bud ectodermam regulates apical ectodermal ridge formation. *Nature* **386**, 366-373.
46.   Lindsell C. E., Shawber, C. J., Boulter, J., and Weinmaster, G. (1995). Jagged: A Mammalian Ligand That Activates Notch 1. *Cell* **80**, 909-917.
47.   Jameson S. C., Hogquist, K. A., and Bevan, M. J. (1995). Positive selection of thymocytes. *Annu. Rev. Immunol.* **13**, 93-126.
48.   Robey E. A., and Fowlkes, B. J. (1994). Selective events in T cell development. *Annu. Rev. Immunol.* **12**, 675-705.
49.   Robey E., Chang, D., Itano, A., Cacano, D., Alexander, H., D., L., Weinmaster, G., and Salmon, P. (1996). An activated form of Notch influences the choice between CD4 and CD8 T cell lineages. *Cell* **87**, 483-492.
50.   Washburn T., Schweigoffer, E., Gridley, T., Chang, D., Fowlkes, B., Cado, D., Salmon, P., and Robey, E. (1997). Notch activity influences the αβ vs. γδ T cell lineage decision. *Cell* **88**, 833-843.
51.   Bigas A., Martin, D. I., and Milner, L. A. (1998). Notch1 and Notch2 inhibit myeloid differentiation in response to different cytokines. *Moll. Cell Biol.* **18**, 2324-2333.
52.   Jones P., May, G., Healey, L., Brown, J., Hoyne, G., Delassus, S., and Enver, T. (1998). Stromal expression of jagged 1 promotes colony formation by fetal haematopoietic progenitor cells. *Blood* **92**, 1505-1511.
53.   Li L., Milner, L. A., Deng, Y., Iwata, M., Banta, A., Graf, L., Marcovina, S., Friedman, C., Trask, B. J., Hood, L., and Torok-Storb, B. (1998). The human homolog of rat Jagged1 expressed by marrow stroma inhibits differentiation of 32D cells through interaction with Notch1. *Immunity* **8**, 43-55.
54.   Varnum-Finney B., Purton, L. E., Yu, M., Brashem-Stein, C., Flowers, D., Staats, S., Moore, K. A., Le Roux, I., Mann, R., Gray, G., Artavanis-Tsakonas, S., and Bernstein, I. D. (1998). The Notch ligand, Jagged-1, influences the development of primitive haematopoietic precursor cells. *Blood* **91**, 4084-4091.
55.   Milner L. A., Bigas, A., Kopan, R., Brashem-Stein, C., Bernstein, I. D., and Martin, D. I. (1996). Inhibition of granulocytic differentiation by mNotch1. *Proc. Natl. Acad. Sci. USA* **93**, 13014-13019.

Acute Lung Injury: From Inflammation to Repair
G.J. Bellingan and G.J. Laurent (Eds.)
IOS Press, 2000

Transgenic and Knockout Mouse Models of Pulmonary Inflammatory Diseases

Mark Griffiths

Adult Intensive Care Unit, Royal Brompton Hospital, Sydney Street, London SW3 6NP, UK

1   Introduction.

The last twenty years has seen explosive progress in the fields of molecular and cell biology. There has been a very real possibility that biochemists would disappear over the horizon leaving physiologists without a means of exploiting the new technology. Since their initial description in 1980 [1], transgenic animal models have to some extent filled this void, providing a powerful tool for examining the biological effects *in vivo* of altering specifically the expression of a single gene. The aim of this article is to highlight the use of transgenic and knockout mice in the investigation of the pathogenesis of pulmonary inflammation; particularly bleomycin induced pulmonary fibrosis (BIPF) an established animal model of human fibrosing alveolitis [2]. The potential of knockout (β6-/-) and transgenic mice is exemplified in this article by recently published investigations by Dean Sheppard at the University of California San Francisco into the role of the integrin alpha v beta 6 (αvβ6) in modulating pulmonary inflammation.

2   Molecular physiology in genetically modified mice.

An enormous amount of genetic information has been uncovered recently by the mapping and sequencing of the Human Genome Project. Alongside this effort, studies in mice have helped to determine the regulation and function of newly identified genes. In a minority of cases established mutations occurring in mouse strains have demonstrated parallels with human disease whose genotype was previously unknown. An example of this phenomenon is the discovery of murine genes that influence obesity, satiety and glucose tolerance, which may lead to the discovery of targets for the treatment of a common human condition [3]. More commonly transgenic or knockout mice are generated as a means of analysing the function of a gene in a mammalian model *in vivo*. Transgenic mice are produced by the permanent insertion of a DNA construct into the mouse genome, whilst a knockout results from the site-specific insertion of DNA into the genome of an embryonic stem cell which disrupts the function of the endogenous gene. In the production of transgenic mice, a DNA construct is injected into the male pronucleus of an oocyte that has been recently fertilised. The transgenic construct usually consists of DNA containing *cis*-active regulatory sequences and a transcriptional "start site" that together control the transcription of downstream DNA. The DNA transgene integrates randomly into the host genome and injected eggs are implanted into a surrogate mother. By contrast, embryonic stem cells carrying knockout or null mutations are injected into a blastocyst and thence transferred to a surrogate mother. *In vitro* study of the differentiation wild-type embryonic stem cells has demonstrated that cell types are produced in a sequence that recapitulates the initial stages of murine embryogenesis [4]. Hence examining the effects of specific mutations in these cell lines may complement developmental studies in knockout mice *in vivo*. The techniques employed to generate transgenic and knockout mice have been extensively reviewed [5].

Having successfully generated transgenic and knockout founder mice, developing useful experimental models requires the breeding of novel lines to homozygosity with painstaking policing of the genotype produced at each generation, and the provision of strain-matched wild type controls. The latter point is particularly pertinent to the study of BIPF in mice, as there is considerable inter-strain variability in the pulmonary inflammatory and fibrotic response to this agent [6,7]. The experiments described below involve either knockout mice that are homozygous for a null mutation affecting a specified gene or transgenic mice expressing a protein that is either not normally present, or if it is, expressing the protein in increased amounts. Valuable information may be gained from such animal's phenotype following over-expression, deletion or inappropriate expression of a targeted gene, however these models may be refined by temporal and/or tissue-directed control of transgenes or knockouts. Temporal control of gene expression or knockout may be required to examine the effects of genetic engineering in the adult, if the mutation confers embryonic lethality or severe developmental defect. An example of an ingenious molecular technique that has been used to overcome this problem is gene expression under the control of a tetracycline-responsive promoter [8] in which tetracycline added to the animal's diet is used to control gene expression. Promoter-enhancer regions from the surfactant protein genes SP-A, -B, -C and CCSP have been used to direct gene expression to the lungs of transgenic mice. SP-C gene expression has been most extensively studied using 3.7kb of 5' sequences from the human SP-C gene (h3.7 SP-C) [9,10]. This region of DNA directed marker gene expression to bronchiolar and type II alveolar epithelial cells in adult transgenic mice and the distal growing tips of the lung bud during foetal development. The level of expression varied significantly between founder lines suggesting that transcription is influenced either by the number of gene copies introduced and/or by the site of transgene insertion into the mouse genome. Alternatively, tissue specific knockout mice can be generated by incorporating two DNA recombinase (Cre) sites (loxP) in a gene of interest into a line and breeding these mice with a second line expressing the bacteriophage recombinase under the control of a promoter such as SP-C. The resulting crosses should have the "floxed" gene deleted in targeted cells following expression of Cre recombinase [11].

Transgenic mice have frequently provided *in vivo* evidence for a biological effect of gene product, which would be difficult to obtain using conventional techniques. Directed expression of human transforming growth factor alpha (h-TGF-α) using the SP-C promoter in mice resulted in h-TGF-α expression exclusively in the distal pulmonary epithelium [12]. The h3.7SP-C-h-TGFα mice developed pulmonary fibrosis of a severity in proportion to the abundance of transgene expression and the founder line. These data suggest that h-TGF-α produced by epithelial cells directly stimulated local mesenchymal cell growth and extracellular collagen deposition. Similarly, transgenic mice expressing tumour necrosis factor alpha (TNF-α) under the control of the SP-C promoter also develop a pulmonary disease that is transmitted to their offspring and which is related to the level of TNF-α mRNA in the lung [13]. Weanling mice developed T lymphocyte predominant alveolitis, which progressed over months to a histological picture resembling human idiopathic pulmonary fibrosis. These data are consistent with a large body of evidence suggesting that

TNF-α plays an important role in the pathogenesis of fibrosing alveolitis [14]. Finally, therapeutic strategies may be tested *in vivo* in the absence of pharmacological agents and without the confounding effects of vectors, such as viruses, required for gene therapy. For example, increased expression of mitochondrial manganese superoxide dismutase under control of the SP-C promoter protects mice against fatal lung injury on exposure to 95% oxygen [15].

Knockout mice may be most useful when alternative means of antagonising a gene product (specific blocking antibodies or peptides) are unavailable or may be used to complement information gained from studies using wild type mice. The data from experiments on knockout mice must be interpreted with the same degree of caution as other models, because there is potential for unpredicted interference with other genes and adaptation to the mutation by other pathways. For example, in a model of complement/neutrophil-dependent lung injury in wild type mice the injury is mediated by reactive oxygen species and is attenuated by catalase. Surprisingly, in NADPH oxidase knockout mice lung injury was equal to that found in wild types and was unaffected by catalase [16]. Subsequent studies suggested that in the knockout mice there had been a switch from the NADPH oxidase system to nitric oxide synthase dependent oxidant production. In other cases murine models of human disease based on similar molecular lesions have deviated significantly from the human condition. The best-studied example is the murine model of cystic fibrosis, in which mutation of the cystic fibrosis transmembrane conductance regulator caused a lethal form of meconium ileus, but little evidence of pancreatic or pulmonary disease [17]. Despite the potential pitfalls and expense of creating a knockout, several unexpected and clinically important observations have already been made. Surprisingly, mice deficient in granulocyte-macrophage colony stimulating factor (GM-CSF) and its' receptor (IL-3/GM-CSF/IL-5 beta c) preserve normal haematopoiesis but demonstrate pulmonary pathology that is indistinguishable from the rare human disease alveolar proteinosis [18,19]. The striking pulmonary pathology in GM-CSF-/- mice is reversed by pulmonary epithelial expression of GM-CSF [20] and improved by adenovirus-mediated pulmonary expression of GM-CSF [21]. IL-3/GM-CSF/IL-5 beta c receptor-deficient mice have been given bone marrow transplants using wild type donor marrow reportedly resulting in resolution of the lung disease [19] or improvement in the proteinosis, but residual pulmonary inflammation [22]. These data not only provide invaluable insight into the mechanisms of a previously poorly understood condition, but also suggest novel therapies for patients with disease that fails to respond to therapeutic lavage. Bone marrow transplant has been suggested as a possible therapy [19] and cases showing a response to GM-CSF have been reported [23].

3   The epithelial cell integrin αvβ6.

Integrins constitute a large family of heterodimeric transmembrane cell surface receptors that recognise as ligands components of the extracellular matrix and other cell's adhesion molecules from the immunoglobulin and cadhedrin families [24]. As adhesion molecules expressed by all cells, integrins play an important role mediating cell adhesion, spreading and migration [25]. For example null mutations of both α6 and β4 integrins are lethal at birth demonstrating widespread epithelial disruption and detachment, because epithelia depend on the constitutive expression of α6β4 to bind laminin 5 a major component of the basement membrane [26]. It has become increasingly evident however, that integrins are used by the cell to determine its' fundamental responses to the immediate environment including survival [27], progression through the cell cycle and differentiation [28]. Furthermore, integrin ligation influences the expression of an increasing list of genes, including matrix metalloproteinases [29], modulators of apoptosis [27], cytokines and growth factors [30]. The basement membranes underlying epithelial cells from α3 knockout mice are highly disorganised, demonstrating a role for this integrin in the structural organisation of the underlying basement membrane [31]. Finally, integrins influence cell behaviour because cells express certain integrins only under specific conditions for example during development, carcinogenesis or when stimulated by cytokines or growth factors [32].

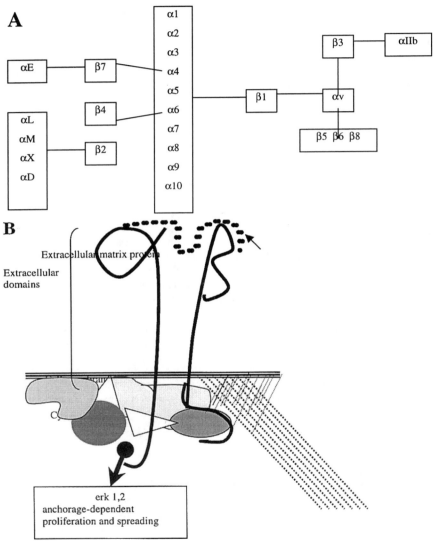

Figure 1. A. Known pairings of integrin subunits. B.A model integrin with attached extracellular matrix protein ligand. The intracellular domains associate with the cytoskeleton and proteins that are involved with signal transduction pathways such as Focal Adhesion Kinase (FAK), Paxicillin, Ras and Src family proteins. Multiple integrins cause cell spreading through interaction with erk 1, 2 (shown).

Integrins, consisting of variable combinations of 17α and 8β subunits, function as cell surface adhesion molecules and as dynamic receptors. The long extracellular domains confer specific ligand binding and the short cytoplasmic domains associate with multimeric protein complexes that are concentrated at sites of cell contact with neighbouring cells or extracellular matrix (Figure 1).

The multimeric complexes contain docking proteins that associate with the cytoskeleton and with effector proteins that are known to initiate and transduce signals mediated by other transmembrane receptor families [33]. Whilst several signalling moieties are known to associate with integrin cytoplasmic tails, the signal transduction pathways that are activated by integrin ligation are as yet poorly understood. Similarly, there is an apparently aimless redundancy of integrin expression. Commonly more than one integrin is expressed which binds to a single matrix ligand; also many integrins whose ligands are not normally present in the basement membrane are constitutively expressed [34]. Clearly there remains a great deal that is not understood about these ubiquitous and pleuripotent cell surface receptors.

In the early 90's Sheppard and co-workers used the homology-based polymerase chain reaction to identify known and novel integrin subunits in airway epithelial cells as part of an investigation into the mechanisms underlying the control of airway inflammation [35]. Three integrin subunits were discovered that participate in the formation of at least four novel integrin heterodimers. The best characterized of these, alpha v beta 6 (αvβ6) [36], is a receptor for the extracellular matrix proteins fibronectin [37], tenascin [38] and vitronectin [25]. Whilst β6 only forms heterodimers with αv, the latter is more promiscuous (Figure 1). αvβ6 appears to be expressed exclusively in terminally differentiated epithelial cells, but is undetectable or scarcely present in normal adult epithelia, except in the secretory phase endometrium. αvβ6 is also highly expressed in the lung, skin and kidney during organogenesis and in human carcinomas [32]. In wounded human skin αvβ6 is expressed in the keratinocytes at the wound edge within a few days of injury, where it persists until soon after wound closure [39]. In lungs of adults for example, αvβ6 is absent from normal airway epithelium but is upregulated in smokers, patients with asthma and in the small airways of patients suffering from fibrosing alveolitis [32, 40]. In a model of acute lung injury in rabbits, αvβ6 mRNA is expressed in alveolar type II cells in a matter of hours after acid instillation [32]. These observations suggest that like its' extracellular matrix protein ligands in skin [40] and lung [41], αvβ6 expression may be induced by inflammation and injury.

Elucidating the functional effects of αvβ6 expression and ligation has proved to be difficult. However, heterologous expression of αvβ6 in a human colon carcinoma cell line (SW480) enhances the proliferative capacity of these cells, both *in vitro* in 3-dimensional collagen gels and *in vivo* in nude mice [42]. This property of αvβ6 correlates with the presence of an 11-amino acid region at the COOH terminus of the β6 cytoplasmic domain. This 11-amino acid sequence is required for the growth stimulatory effect, but not for other functions of the β6 cytoplasmic domain, such as promoting cell adhesion and focal contact localization [42]. In the absence of blocking antibodies and peptides, mice homozygous for a null mutation in the gene encoding the β6 subunit were generated to examine the effects of αvβ6 *in vivo* [43]. Beta 6 knockout mice (β6-/-) had obvious juvenile baldness at the back of their heads and necks associated with local infiltration of macrophages in the dermis. Similarly, accumulated lymphocytes were evident around conducting airways and in the lung parenchyma foamy macrophages were evident in β6-/- mice but not in wild type controls. All lymphocyte subsets were increased in single cell preparations from the lungs of β6-/- mice, including T cells expressing the interleukin 2 (IL-2) receptor CD25, which is a marker of lymphocyte activation. Beta 6-/- mice demonstrated corresponding airway hyperresponsiveness to acetylcholine, a hallmark of asthma. These results gave the first indication that the epithelial integrin αvβ6 participates in the modulation of local epithelial inflammation [43]. This impression was reinforced when the same group generated transgenic mice constitutively expressing the human β6 subunit under the control of h3.7SP-C in alveolar type II cells and bronchiolar epithelial [44]. Expression of this transgene largely inhibited the activation and the numerical increase in airspace lymphocytes and macrophages observed in β6-/- mice. In the genetically mixed mice used for this study, airway eosinophilia was identified as an additional effect of β6 inactivation, which was also partially inhibited by limited expression of the human transgene. These results definitively identified a role for distal lung epithelial αvβ6 expression in down-regulating pulmonary inflammation [44]. A possible interpretation of these observations is illustrated below (Figure 2). Hence, the pathway is initiated by mild injury or trauma, for the skin being picked up by one's murine mother by the scruff of the neck and for the airway inhalation of irritant particles. Epithelial cells are induced to express αvβ6 on the cell's surface and a provisional extracellular matrix containing ligands for αvβ6 is formed. Ligation of the integrin is proposed to have a negative feedback effect on the cell's inflammatory response to injury. Epithelia lacking the ability to express αvβ6 would therefore respond to subclinical injury by inducing exaggerated and prolonged inflammation.

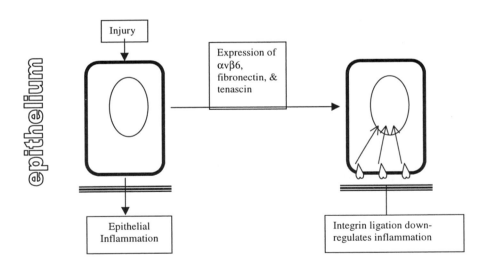

Figure 2. Proposed model demonstrating the anti-inflammatory effect of αvβ6 receptor binding with its' extracellular matrix ligands fibronectin and tenascin, following induction by injury.

4   Bleomycin induced pulmonary fibrosis.

The role of αvβ6 in modulating pulmonary inflammation was investigated further by examining the effects of intratracheal bleomycin on knockout and strain-matched wild type mice. Bleomycin is a naturally occurring chemotherapeutic agent, which as a side effect causes acute lung injury and alveolitis that progresses to pulmonary fibrosis both in patients being treated for cancer [45] and in animal models [2]. Bleomycin binds and disrupts DNA by strand scission requiring oxidation [46] and initiates apoptosis [47].

Predominantly pulmonary side effects may occur because bleomycin is concentrated in pulmonary epithelial and endothelial cells. The pathogenesis of pulmonary fibrosis has been much studied and recently reviewed [48,49], however the questions (a) why the inflammatory response is self-perpetuating after a single exposure to bleomycin, and (b) why the resultant inflammation leads to healing by fibrosis, remain unanswered. Most work has concentrated on the role of inflammatory and fibrogenic mediators expressed by activated lymphocytes and macrophages, the cell types that dominate the pulmonary inflammatory response after the first few days following bleomycin administration. Relatively little attention has been paid to alveolar epithelial cells that have been largely considered as victims of injury and bystanders in the ensuing fibrosis mediated by mesenchymal cells, that proliferate and lay down excessive extracellular collagen matrix. It should be remembered however that pulmonary epithelial cells secrete a large number of pro-inflammatory cytokines [50]. Furthermore, the process of optimal healing after lung injury depends on type II alveolar cells proliferation and spreading over the denuded alveolar membrane to restore the type I cell population and normal alveolar architecture [51].

Five days after tracheal instillation of bleomycin, in the presence of an acute inflammatory infiltrate including granulocytes, the permeability of alveolar-capillary membrane is increased causing pulmonary oedema. The inflammatory exudate has peaked by 15 days, with lymphocytes and macrophages predominating. Pulmonary fibrosis is evident histologically and biochemically after two weeks and increases steadily until at least 60 days after a single bleomycin exposure (personal observations). Predictably, apoptosis in murine bronchiolar and alveolar epithelium has been demonstrated within a day of bleomycin administration, but there was also DNA fragmentation (apoptosis) and smearing (necrosis) in lung tissue in the second week [52]. Associated with the latter, Fas mRNA was upregulated in alveolar epithelial cells and Fas ligand mRNA was expressed in lymphocytes in the inflamed interstitium. This suggests a possible mechanism for on-going epithelial damage, which may be an important determinant of healing by fibrosis [53]. T lymphocytes that are recruited to the injured lung appear to play a major role in BIPF [54,55], but recent evidence suggests that BIPF can occur in their absence [56]. Macrophages are also recruited to the lung after bleomycin administration and produce a variety of cytokines and growth factors that are pro-inflammatory, and others that stimulate fibroblast proliferation and collagen synthesis [57,58]. TNF-α and IL-1 are examples of pro-inflammatory macrophage derived cytokines that have been implicated in the pathogenesis of BIPF. TNF-α but not IL-1 mRNA is found in the lungs of bleomycin treated mice. However, both anti-TNF-α antibodies [14] and IL-1 receptor antagonist block BIPF in murine models. Whilst many other cell types and secreted products have been shown to play roles in the inflammation and healing by fibrosis that characterises bleomycin induced lung damage, an exhaustive review is beyond the scope of this article.

5   Transforming growth factor beta.

Transforming growth factor beta (TGF-β), of all the growth factors and cytokines associated with BIPF perhaps is the most likely to play an essential role as the final common pathway leading to fibrosis. The TGF-β family consists of three closely related isoforms (TGF-β1, 2 and 3), that are prototypes of the larger TGF-β superfamily. *In vitro*, TGF-βs exert nearly identical effects that can be grouped into three areas: modulation of inflammatory cell function, growth inhibition and differentiation, and control of extracellular matrix production. Studies of animal models [59] as well as human specimens [60] strongly suggest that TGF-β is important in the pathogenesis of several diseases, including pulmonary fibrotic conditions [61]. Specifically, BIPF in mice may be attenuated by the systemic administration of antibodies to both TGF-β-1 and TGF-β-2 immediately after injury [62]. Gene knockouts have helped elucidate TGF-β's roles and the differences among the isoforms. TGF-β-1 knockout mice develop diffuse mononuclear cell infiltrates that prove lethal within a few weeks from birth [63,64]. By contrast, TGF-β-2 and TGF-β-3 knockout mice display only developmental defects [65,66].

The TGF-βs are secreted as complexes composed of three proteins derived from two genes. Each TGF-β gene encodes a procytokine consisting of a C-terminal TGF-β sequence and a larger N-terminal region that, after processing, forms a protein called Latency Associated Peptide (LAP). LAP-β1 and LAP-β3 contain arginine-glycine-aspartic acid (RGD) amino acid sequences, which are also binding site motifs in ligands for a subset of integrins. LAP-β1 can bind effectively to one such integrin, (αvβ1), but the functional role of LAP-integrin interactions is not known [67]. LAP and TGF-β remain non-covalently associated, and in this configuration TGF-β is unable to bind to receptors and is thus latent. In most cases, the complex of LAP and TGF-β (the small latent complex, SLC) is joined by latent TGF-β binding protein-1 (LTBP-1), a matrix protein with sequence similarity to the fibrillins. LAP is disulfide-linked to a specific cystine-rich domain of LTBP [68, 69], and the complex of all three proteins is called the large latent complex (LLC). Latent TGF-β can be linked by LTBP to binding sites in the extracellular matrix [70]. The mechanisms involved in activating latent TGF-β are not fully understood, but recently there has been important progress in this area [71]. Plasmin can activate latent TGF in cell culture [72], but plasminogen knockout mice display none of the pathologic features of TGF-β knockout mice [73], suggesting that plasmin is unlikely to be the only molecule activating TGF-β. Reactive oxygen species can activate TGF-β *in vitro*, and radiation treatment also appears to be able to activate TGF-β *in vivo* via this mechanism [74]. Thrombospondin (TSP)-1 can activate TGF-β by binding to a defined site on LAP and inducing a conformational change in the latent complex; TGF-β is then bound to TSP-1 in an active state [75]. Similar patterns of inflammation are exhibited by TGF-β-1 and TSP-1 knockout mice suggesting that TSP-1 is a major activator of TGF-β-1 *in vivo*. However, the inflammatory changes in the TSP-1 knockout mice are less severe than those observed in TGF-β-1 knockout mice [76]; these data again suggest that there are multiple and probably overlapping mechanisms of TGF-β activation.

6   Bleomycin induced pulmonary fibrosis in mice lacking epithelial αvβ6.

Analysis of the hydroxyproline content of lungs from wild type and β6-/- mice 30 to 60 days after intratracheal administration of bleomycin demonstrated that the knockout mice were dramatically protected against pulmonary fibrosis [77]. Histological examination of lungs throughout the month after bleomycin dosing suggested that the β6-/- mice, experienced an acute alveolitis but that the degree to which healing restored normal lung architecture was greater than that seen in the wild type controls. Examination of the pulmonary inflammatory cell infiltrates by flow cytometry suggested that recruitment and activation of lymphocytes and macrophages was not deficient in β6-/- mice. These data confirmed the presence of greater numbers of lymphocytes and macrophages in the lungs of untreated knockout mice as had previously been seen [43]. In wild type mice αvβ6 expression was upregulated in areas of lung with acute alveolitis, however no change in TGF-β expression was demonstrable at any time after bleomycin in wild type or knockout mice.

Given the failure of a TGF-β-dependent process (BIPF) in β6-/- mice and similarities between the spontaneous inflammatory lesions in TGF-β-/- and β6-/- mice, it was proposed that the β6-/- phenotype was caused by impaired expression of activated

TGF-β as had previously been observed in TSP-1 mice [76]. It was demonstrated that LAP-β1 is a ligand for αvβ6, as it is for other integrins [67], binding at the RGD site located near the C-terminus. Furthermore, several cell lines expressing αvβ6 activated endogenous latent TGFβ-1 when co-cultured with TGF-β-sensitive reporter cells in the absence of a wide range of proteases and molecules, such as plasmin and TSP-1, which have previously been shown to mediate activation. A possible mechanism of non-proteolytic activation of TGFβ-1, would involve a critical conformation change in LAP leading directly to activation of the latent complex [78]. Finally, not only was ligation of LAP-containing latent TGFβ-1 complexes associated with TGFβ-1 activation, but the authors demonstrated induction of phosphorylation of FAK and paxillin, proteins that have been implicated in integrin signal transduction (Figure 1). This finding raises the possibility that locally produced latent TGFβ-1 complexes could influence epithelial cell behaviour through integrin ligation.

These experiments highlight the central role of TGFβ-1in modulating inflammation and reveal unexpected effects of αvβ6 integrin expression and ligation. TGFβ-1 induces αvβ6 expression [79], as well as inducing its' own expression [80]. Both positive feedback effects suggest the existence of potent antagonists of TGF-β activation and expression that are currently poorly understood, but which may be important therapeutic targets in the control of fibrotic diseases.

7   Summary.

Genetically altered mice have become invaluable tools in biomedical research allowing workers to examine the effects of targeted gene manipulation *in vivo*. The use of murine models of pulmonary inflammation and fibrosis have been discussed, with particular reference to recent investigations into the roles of TGF-β and the epithelial integrin αvβ6 in the pathogenesis of BIPF. Observations made in mice with engineered null mutations of the TGFβ-1 and β6 subunit genes have helped to reveal a novel mechanism of TGFβ-1 activation involving a critical conformational change induced by binding of the latent TGFβ-1 complex to αvβ6.

References.

1.   Gordon JW, Scangos GA, Plotkin DJ, Barbosa JA, Ruddle FH. (1980) Genetic transformation of mouse embryos by microinjection of purified DNA. *Proc. Natl. Acad. Sci. U S A*; **77**: 7380-4.
2.   Adamson IY, Bowden DH. (1974) The pathogenesis of bleomycin-induced pulmonary fibrosis in mice. *Am J Pathol* **77**: 185-97.
3.   Levine AS, Billington CJ. (1998) Obesity: progress through genetic manipulation. *Curr Biol*; **8**: R251-2.
4.   Weiss MJ, Orkin SH. (1996) In vitro differentiation of murine embryonic stem cells. New approaches to old problems. *J Clin Invest;* **97**: 591-5.
5.   Rossant J, Nagy A. (1995) Genome engineering: the new mouse genetics. *Nat Med*; **1**: 592-4.
6.   Haston CK, Amos CI, King TM, Travis EL. (1996) Inheritance of susceptibility to bleomycin-induced pulmonary fibrosis in the mouse. *Cancer Res.;* **56**: 2596-601.
7.   Schrier DJ, Kunkel RG, Phan SH. (1983) The role of strain variation in murine bleomycin-induced pulmonary fibrosis. *Am Rev Respir Dis;* **127**: 63-6.
8.   Furth PA, St Onge L, Boger H, *et al.* (1994) Temporal control of gene expression in transgenic mice by a tetracycline-responsive promoter. *Proc. Natl. Acad. Sci. U S A;* **91**: 9302-6.
9.   Glasser SW, Korfhagen TR, Wert SE, *et al.* (1991) Genetic element from human surfactant protein SP-C gene confers bronchiolar-alveolar cell specificity in transgenic mice. *Am J Physiol;* **261**: L349-56.

10.   Korfhagen TR, Glasser SW, Wert SE, *et al.* (1990) Cis-acting sequences from a human surfactant protein gene confer pulmonary-specific gene expression in transgenic mice. *Proc. Natl. Acad. Sci. U S A;* **87:** 6122-6.

11.   Lakso M, Sauer B, Mosinger B, Jr., *et al.* (1992) Targeted oncogene activation by site-specific recombination in transgenic mice. *Proc. Natl. Acad. Sci. U S A;* **89:** 6232-6.

12.   Korfhagen TR, Swantz RJ, Wert SE, *et al.* (1994) Respiratory epithelial cell expression of human transforming growth factor-alpha induces lung fibrosis in transgenic mice. *J Clin Invest;* **93:** 1691-9.

13.   Miyazaki Y, Araki K, Vesin C, *et al.* (1995) Expression of a tumor necrosis factor-alpha transgene in murine lung causes lymphocytic and fibrosing alveolitis. A mouse model of progressive pulmonary fibrosis. *J Clin Invest;* **96:** 250-9.

14.   Piguet PF, Collart MA, Grau GE, Kapanci Y, Vassalli P. (1989) Tumor necrosis factor/cachectin plays a key role in bleomycin-induced pneumopathy and fibrosis. *J. Exp. Med. ;* **170:** 655-63.

15.   Wispe JR, Warner BB, Clark JC, *et al.* (1992) Human Mn-superoxide dismutase in pulmonary epithelial cells of transgenic mice confers protection from oxygen injury. *J. Biol. Chem.;* **267:** 23937-41.

16.   Kubo H, Morgenstern D, Quinian WM, Ward PA, Dinauer MC, Doerschuk CM. (1996) Preservation of complement-induced lung injury in mice with deficiency of NADPH oxidase. *J Clin Invest;* **97:** 2680-4.

17.   Clarke LL, Grubb BR, Gabriel SE, Smithies O, Koller BH, Boucher RC. (1992) Defective epithelial chloride transport in a gene-targeted mouse model of cystic fibrosis. *Science;* **257:** 1125-8.

18.   Dranoff G, Crawford AD, Sadelain M, *et al.* (1994) Involvement of granulocyte-macrophage colony-stimulating factor in pulmonary homeostasis. *Science;* **264:** 713-6.

19.   Nishinakamura R, Wiler R, Dirksen U, *et al.* (1996) The pulmonary alveolar proteinosis in granulocyte macrophage colony- stimulating factor/interleukins 3/5 beta c receptor-deficient mice is reversed by bone marrow transplantation. *J. Exp. Med. ;* **183:** 2657-62.

20.   Huffman JA, Hull WM, Dranoff G, Mulligan RC, Whitsett JA. (1996) Pulmonary epithelial cell expression of GM-CSF corrects the alveolar proteinosis in GM-CSF-deficient mice. *J Clin Invest;* **97:** 649-55.

21.   Zsengeller ZK, Reed JA, Bachurski CJ, *et al.* (1998) Adenovirus-mediated granulocyte-macrophage colony-stimulating factor improves lung pathology of pulmonary alveolar proteinosis in granulocyte-macrophage colony-stimulating factor-deficient mice. *Hum Gene Ther;* **9:** 2101-9.

22.   Cooke KR, Nishinakamura R, Martin TR, *et al.* (1997) Persistence of pulmonary pathology and abnormal lung function in IL- 3/GM-CSF/IL-5 beta c receptor-deficient mice despite correction of alveolar proteinosis after BMT. *Bone Marrow Transplant;* **20:** 657-62.

23.   Seymour JF, Dunn AR, Vincent JM, Presneill JJ, Pain MC. (1996) Efficacy of granulocyte-macrophage colony-stimulating factor in acquired alveolar proteinosis. *N. Engl. J. Med. ;* **335:** 1924-5.

24.   Hynes RO. (1987) Integrins: a family of cell surface receptors. *Cell;* **48:** 549-54.

25.   Huang X, Wu J, Spong S, Sheppard D. (1998) The integrin alphavbeta6 is critical for keratinocyte migration on both its known ligand, fibronectin, and on vitronectin. J Cell Sci; **111:** 2189-95.

26.   van der Neut R, Krimpenfort P, Calafat J, Niessen CM, Sonnenberg A. (1996) Epithelial detachment due to absence of hemidesmosomes in integrin beta 4 null mice. *Nat Genet;* **13:** 366-9

27.   Boudreau N, Sympson CJ, Werb Z, Bissell MJ. (1995) Suppression of ICE and apoptosis in mammary epithelial cells by extracellular matrix. *Science;* **267:** 891-3.

28.   Ronnov-Jessen L, Petersen OW, Bissell MJ. (1996) Cellular changes involved in conversion of normal to malignant breast: importance of the stromal reaction. *Physiol Rev;* **76:** 69-125.

29.   Werb Z, Tremble PM, Behrendtsen O, Crowley E, Damsky CH. (1989) Signal transduction through the fibronectin receptor induces collagenase and stromelysin gene expression. *J Cell Biol;* **109:** 877-89.

30.   Miyake S, Yagita H, Maruyama T, Hashimoto H, Miyasaka N, Okumura K. (1993) Beta 1 integrin-mediated interaction with extracellular matrix proteins regulates cytokine gene expression in synovial fluid cells of rheumatoid arthritis patients. *J. Exp. Med. ;* **177:** 863-8.

31.   DiPersio CM, Hodivala-Dilke KM, Jaenisch R, Kreidberg JA, Hynes RO. (1997) alpha3beta1 Integrin is required for normal development of the epidermal basement membrane. *J Cell Biol;* **137:** 729-42.

32.   Breuss JM, Gillett N, Lu L, Sheppard D, Pytela R. (1993) Restricted distribution of integrin beta 6 mRNA in primate epithelial tissues. *J Histochem Cytochem;* **41:** 1521-7.

33.   Clark EA, Brugge JS. (1995) Integrins and signal transduction pathways: the road taken. *Science;* **268:** 233-9.

34.   Sheppard D. (1998) Airway epithelial integrins: why so many? *Am J Respir Cell Moll Biol;* **19:** 349-51.

35. Sheppard D, Erle D, Busk M, Pytela R. (1992) Identification of novel airway epithelial integrins using the homology- based polymerase chain reaction. *Chest;* **101:** 49S.
36. Sheppard D, Rozzo C, Starr L, Quaranta V, Erle DJ, Pytela R. (1990) Complete amino acid sequence of a novel integrin beta subunit (beta 6) identified in epithelial cells using the polymerase chain reaction. *J. Biol. Chem.;* **265:** 11502-7.
37. Busk M, Pytela R, Sheppard D. (1992) Characterization of the integrin alpha v beta 6 as a fibronectin- binding protein. *J. Biol. Chem.;* **267:** 5790-6.
38. Prieto AL, Edelman GM, Crossin KL. (1993) Multiple integrins mediate cell attachment to cytotactin/tenascin. *Proc. Natl. Acad. Sci. U S A;* **90**10154-8.
39. Haapasalmi K, Zhang K, Tonnesen M, *et al.* (1996) Keratinocytes in human wounds express alpha v beta 6 integrin. *J Invest Dermatol;* **106:** 42-8.
40. Weinacker A, Ferrando R, Elliott M, Hogg J, Balmes J, Sheppard D. (1995) Distribution of integrins alpha v beta 6 and alpha 9 beta 1 and their known ligands, fibronectin and tenascin, in human airways. *Am J Respir Cell Moll Biol;* **12:** 547-56.
41. Harrison JH, Jr., Hoyt DG, Lazo JS. (1989) Acute pulmonary toxicity of bleomycin: DNA scission and matrix protein mRNA levels in bleomycin-sensitive and -resistant strains of mice. *Moll Pharmacol;* **36:** 231-8.
42. Agrez M, Chen A, Cone RI, Pytela R, Sheppard D. (1994) The alpha v beta 6 integrin promotes proliferation of colon carcinoma cells through a unique region of the beta 6 cytoplasmic domain. *J Cell Biol;* **127:** 547-56.
43. Huang XZ, Wu JF, Cass D, *et al.* (1996) Inactivation of the integrin beta 6 subunit gene reveals a role of epithelial integrins in regulating inflammation in the lung and skin. *J Cell Biol;* **133:** 921-8.
44. Huang X, Wu J, Zhu W, Pytela R, Sheppard D. (1998) Expression of the human integrin beta6 subunit in alveolar type II cells and bronchiolar epithelial cells reverses lung inflammation in beta6 knockout mice. *Am J Respir Cell Moll Biol;* **19:** 636-42.
45. Ginsberg SJ, Comis RL. (1982) The pulmonary toxicity of antineoplastic agents. *Semin. Oncol.;* **9:** 34-51.
46. Hecht SM. (1986) DNA strand scission by activated bleomycin group antibiotics. *Fed Proc;* **45:** 2784-91.
47. Muller M, Wilder S, Bannasch D, *et al.* (1998) p53 activates the CD95 (APO-1/Fas) gene in response to DNA damage by anticancer drugs. *J. Exp. Med. ;* **188:** 2033-45.
48. Kumar RK, Lykke AW. (1995) Messages and handshakes: cellular interactions in pulmonary fibrosis. *Pathology;* **27:** 18-26.
49. Bienkowski RS, Gotkin MG. (1995) Control of collagen deposition in mammalian lung. *Proc. Soc. Exp. Biol. Med. ;* **209:** 118-40.
50. Sheppard D. Epithelial integrins. Bioessays 1996; 18:655-60.
51. Witschi H. (1991) Role of the epithelium in lung repair. *Chest;* **99:** 22S-25S.
52. Hagimoto N, Kuwano K, Nomoto Y, Kunitake R, Hara N. (1997) Apoptosis and expression of Fas/Fas ligand mRNA in bleomycin-induced pulmonary fibrosis in mice. *Am J Respir Cell Moll Biol;* **16:** 91-101.
53. Ortiz LA, Moroz K, Liu JY, *et al.* (1998) Alveolar macrophage apoptosis and TNF-alpha, but not p53, expression correlate with murine response to bleomycin. *Am J Physiol;* **275:** L1208-18.
54. Schrier DJ, Phan SH. (1984) Modulation of bleomycin-induced pulmonary fibrosis in the BALB/c mouse by cyclophosphamide-sensitive T cells. *Am J Pathol;* **116:** 270-8.
55. Sharma SK, MacLean JA, Pinto C, Kradin RL. (1996) The effect of an anti-CD3 monoclonal antibody on bleomycin-induced lymphokine production and lung injury. *Am. J. Respir. Crit. Care Med.;* **154:** 193-200.
56. Helene M, Lake-Bullock V, Zhu J, Hao H, Cohen DA, Kaplan AM. (1999) T cell independence of bleomycin-induced pulmonary fibrosis. *J Leukoc Biol;* **65:** 187-95.
57. Rappolee DA, Werb Z. (1992) Macrophage-derived growth factors. *Curr Top Microbiol Immunol;* **181:** 87-140.
58. Henke C, Marineili W, Jessurun J, *et al.* (1993) Macrophage production of basic fibroblast growth factor in the fibroproliferative disorder of alveolar fibrosis after lung injury. *Am J Pathol;* **143:** 1189-99.
59. Sime PJ, Xing Z, Graham FL, Csaky KG, Gauldie J. (1997) Adenovector-mediated gene transfer of active transforming growth factor- beta1 induces prolonged severe fibrosis in rat lung. *J Clin Invest;* **100:** 768-76.
60. Broekelmann TJ, Limper AH, Colby TV, McDonald JA. (1991) Transforming growth factor beta 1 is present at sites of extracellular matrix gene expression in human pulmonary fibrosis. *Proc. Natl. Acad. Sci. U S A;* **88:** 6642-6.
61. Border WA, Noble NA. (1994) Transforming growth factor beta in tissue fibrosis. *N. Engl. J. Med.;* **331:** 1286-92.

62.   Giri SN, Hyde DM, Hollinger MA. (1993) Effect of antibody to transforming growth factor beta on bleomycin induced accumulation of lung collagen in mice. *Thorax;* **48:** 959-66.

63.   Shull MM, Ormsby I, Kier AB, *et al.* (1992) Targeted disruption of the mouse transforming growth factor-beta 1 gene results in multifocal inflammatory disease. *Nature*; **359:** 693-9.

64.   Kulkarni AB, Karlsson S. (1993) Transforming growth factor-beta 1 knockout mice. A mutation in one cytokine gene causes a dramatic inflammatory disease. *Am J Pathol;* **143:** 3-9.

65.   Sanford LP, Ormsby I, Gittenberger-de Groot AC, *et al.* (1997) TGFbeta2 knockout mice have multiple developmental defects that are non- overlapping with other TGF-beta knockout phenotypes. *Development;* **124:** 2659-70.

66.   Kaartinen V, Voncken JW, Shuler C, *et al.* (1995) Abnormal lung development and cleft palate in mice lacking TGF-beta 3 indicates defects of epithelial-mesenchymal interaction. *Nat Genet;* **11:** 415-21.

67.   Munger JS, Harpel JG, Giancotti FG, Rifkin DB. (1998) Interactions between growth factors and integrins: latent forms of transforming growth factor-beta are ligands for the integrin alphavbeta1. *Moll Biol Cell;* **9:** 2627-38.

68.   Saharinen J, Taipale J, Keski-Oja J. (1996) Association of the small latent transforming growth factor-beta with an eight cysteine repeat of its binding protein LTBP-1. *Embo. J.;* **15:** 245-53.

69.   Gleizes PE, Beavis RC, Mazzieri R, Shen B, Rifkin DB. (1996) Identification and characterization of an eight-cysteine repeat of the latent transforming growth factor-beta binding protein-1 that mediates bonding to the latent transforming growth factor-beta1. *J. Biol. Chem.;* **271:** 29891-6.

70.   Taipale J, Saharinen J, Hedman K, Keski-Oja J. (1996) Latent transforming growth factor-beta 1 and its binding protein are components of extracellular matrix microfibrils. *J Histochem Cytochem;* **44:** 875-89.

71.   Gleizes PE, Munger JS, Nunes I, *et al.* (1997) TGF-beta latency: biological significance and mechanisms of activation. *Stem Cells;* **15:** 190-7.

72.   Sato Y, Tsuboi R, Lyons R, Moses H, Rifkin DB. (1990) Characterization of the activation of latent TGF-beta by co-cultures of endothelial cells and pericytes or smooth muscle cells: a self- regulating system. *J Cell Biol*; **111:** 757-63.

73.   Carmeliet P, Kieckens L, Schoonjans L, *et al.* (1993) Plasminogen activator inhibitor-1 gene-deficient mice. I. Generation by homologous recombination and characterization. *J Clin Invest;* **92:** 2746-55.

74.   Barcellos-Hoff MH, Derynck R, Tsang ML, Weatherbee JA. (1994) Transforming growth factor-beta activation in irradiated murine mammary gland. *J Clin Invest;* 93: 892-9.

75.   Schultz-Cherry S, Chen H, Mosher DF, *et al.* (1995) Regulation of transforming growth factor-beta activation by discrete sequences of thrombospondin 1. *J. Biol. Chem.;* **270:** 7304-10.

76.   Crawford SE, Stellmach V, Murphy-Ullrich JE, *et al.* (1998) Thrombospondin-1 is a major activator of TGF-beta1 in vivo. *Cell;* **93:** 1159-70.

77.   Munger JS, Huang X, Kawakatsu H, *et al.* (1999) The integrin alpha v beta 6 binds and activates latent TGF beta 1: a mechanism for regulating pulmonary inflammation and fibrosis. *Cell;* **96:** 319-28.

78.   McMahon GA, Dignam JD, Gentry LE. (1996) Structural characterization of the latent complex between transforming growth factor beta 1 and beta 1-latency-associated peptide. *Biochem J;* **313:** 343-51.

79.   Wang A, Yokosaki Y, Ferrando R, Balmes J, Sheppard D. (1996) Differential regulation of airway epithelial integrins by growth factors. *Am J Respir Cell Moll* Biol; **15:** 664-72.

80.   Van Obberghen-Schilling E, Roche NS, Flanders KC, Sporn MB, Roberts AB. (1988) Transforming growth factor beta 1 positively regulates its own expression in normal and transformed cells. *J. Biol. Chem.;* **263:** 7741-6.

The Fibroproliferative Response to Acute Lung Injury

Richard P. Marshall, Geoffrey J Bellingan and Geoffrey J Laurent

Centre for Cardiopulmonary Biochemistry & Respiratory Medicine
Royal Free University College Medical School, Rayne Institute
University Street, London WC1E 6JJ, UK

1   Introduction.

ARDS represents a severe and rapid form of acute lung injury that continues to be associated with a high mortality rate [1, 2]. The full repertoire of repair responses are brought into play, all of which are facilitated by a process of decompartmentalisation in which fluid, proteins and cells move or migrate between the vascular, interstitial, alveolar and pleural spaces (Figure 1). The resulting fibrosis is histologically and biochemically similar to that seen in other more chronic forms of interstitial lung disease [3] however, much less is known of the mediators and cellular events occurring in ARDS.

In this chapter we will outline factors believed to play key roles in the development of lung fibrosis and discuss their possible involvement in ARDS. We will also examine the timing of the onset of fibroproliferation, contrasting accepted beliefs with newer understanding of these processes. In addition, a number of elements more specific to ARDS and its therapy will be discussed as potential influences on the fibrotic response. Understanding such processes in the apparently chaotic milieu that exists in the lungs of ARDS patients is an important challenge to respiratory biology but is likely to have enormous relevance to lung injury and repair in a number of disease settings.

2   Fibroproliferation in ARDS: the players.

Interstitial and intra-alveolar fibrosis are hallmarks of the more advanced stages of ARDS and are characterised by the abnormal and excessive deposition of extracellular matrix proteins, in particular collagen. The decrease in pulmonary compliance and progressive hypoxia resulting from fibrotic change leads to ventilator dependence. As a result, progressive fibrosis is a direct cause of respiratory death in up to 40% of patients [4, 5] but is also an indirect cause of death due to nosocomial infection and progressive multi-organ failure in up to 70% of patients dying from ARDS [6].

At the onset of ARDS, the local environment in all lung compartments is radically altered. The movement of proteinacious fluid and cells from the circulation is coupled with the activation of resident cells. A complex interaction between epithelial, endothelial, mesenchymal and inflammatory cells ensues with intense signalling via chemical mediators and the direct influence of the oxidative, mechanical and osmotic environment. Some of the key cell types and their activation are discussed below.

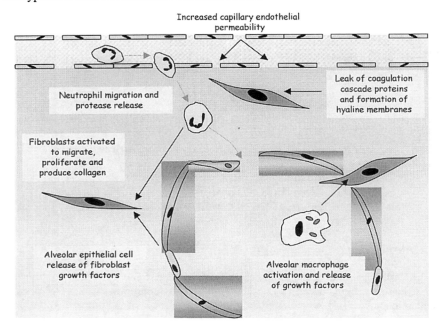

Figure 1. Mechanisms of fibroproliferation in ARDS.

2.1   Endothelial cells.

Activation of the microvascular endothelium is one of the earliest events in ARDS. An increase in permeability leads to profound flooding of the alveolar and interstitial space with proteinacious fluid. This low-pressure pulmonary oedema provides a potent source of profibrotic mediators including circulating chemokines and proteins of the coagulation cascade (see following Chapter). Moreover, changes in the expression of specific adhesion molecules on the microvascular endothelium (e.g. Selectins, CD11b/18) [7] and chemotactic stimuli (e.g. IL-8 and IL-4) [8] lead to an early and persistent accumulation of neutrophils in the lung (see below). Signalling between the capillary endothelium and interstitial fibroblasts could also be an important mechanism in the pathogenesis of ARDS and deserves further attention.

2.2   Inflammatory cells.

Neutrophils and other inflammatory cells entering the pulmonary interstitium and alveolar space release a host of pro-inflammatory cytokines. TNF-α, IL-1β, IL-2, IL-4, IL-6, IL-8 [8] are all elevated within 24 hours of the onset of acute lung injury and persist in non-survivors. In addition to their pro-inflammatory activity, these cytokines are also potentially fibrogenic. TNF-α, for example stimulates lung fibroblast collagen synthesis [9]. Furthermore, TNF-α gene expression is also increased in an animal model of fibrotic lung injury induced by bleomycin [10] and over expression can induce interstitial pulmonary fibrosis in mice [11].

Alveolar macrophages are also an important source of profibrotic cytokines including TGF β and Insulin-like growth factor-1 [12]. IGF-1 stimulates collagen synthesis [13], and is at least partly responsible for the fibroblast mitogenic activity observed in bronchoalveolar lavage fluid of patients with systemic sclerosis [14]. Alveolar macrophages are increased in animal models of acute lung injury and in ARDS BALF [15-17], although the neutrophil is the predominant cell type in absolute terms [18].

Mast cells are increased in the BALF of patients with progressive ARDS [19]. Although increases in collagen deposition appear to precede mast cell accumulation, they could contribute to the activation of fibroblasts by the release of their granule contents. In particular, the mast cell product, tryptase is mitogenic for fibroblasts *in vitro* [20].

2.3   Epithelial cells.

Even in the absence of a direct injury to the lung (e.g.: aspiration or inhalational injury), type I alveolar epithelial cell necrosis together with a proliferation of type II cells is seen in patients with ARDS. The loss of an intact epithelial basement membrane allows the migration of inflammatory cells and fibroblasts into the alveolar space. The importance of maintaining epithelial cell layer integrity is suggested by observations in a number of animal models in which potent growth factors for epithelial cells such as keratinocyte growth factor and hepatocyte growth factor effectively attenuate lung injury and the subsequent development of fibrosis when administered before the injurious agent [21, 22]. Furthermore in BAL of patients with ALI the levels of hepatocyte growth factor, but not keratinocyte growth factor are significantly elevated within the first 48 hours after injury [23]. Epithelial cells, once activated may also contribute directly to the fibrotic response, via cytokine signalling. For example, our laboratory has previously shown that IGF-1, released by epithelial cells is an important mitogen for lung fibroblasts *in vitro* [24]. In addition, the epithelial layer plays an important role in the clearance of oedema fluid from the alveolar space and thus the resolution of ARDS.

2.4   Fibroblasts.

The fibroblast represents approximately 40% of pulmonary cells and is the major producer of collagen in the lung although endothelial cells, epithelial cells, alveolar type II cells and smooth muscle cells are also capable of synthesising these proteins. An increase in fibroblast number has been reported in both animal models of pulmonary fibrosis and in man [25]. A number factors have been shown to either stimulate or inhibit fibroblast activation including the autocrine and paracrine action of soluble polypeptide mediators. These cytokines appear to have an important role in the control of fibroblast activity *in vitro,* and have been implicated in the pathogenesis of pulmonary fibrosis in both animal models and in humans.

3   Profibrotic cytokines in the lung.

Profibrotic factors could increase collagen deposition in the lung by stimulating fibroblasts and other collagen producing cells to migrate, proliferate or produce excess collagen via a direct action on those cells or by stimulating the autocrine production of other profibrotic mediators. Transforming growth factor β (TGFβ) is one potent stimulator of collagen production, secreted by alveolar macrophages and fibroblasts themselves, and exemplifies the variety of mechanisms by which cytokine-mediated control of collagen turnover can occur [26–28]. It increases procollagen gene transcription [29, 30], increases mRNA stability [29], decreases the intracellular degradation of collagen [27] and decreases the extracellular degradation of collagen by inhibiting collagenase production and stimulating the production of metalloprotease inhibitors [31, 32]. TGFβ mRNA and protein levels are increased in animal models [33, 34] and in patients with pulmonary fibrosis [35, 36]. At low concentrations TGFβ is also a mitogen for fibroblasts [37]. *In vivo*, the transient over expression of active TGFβ in rat lung resulted in a fibrotic response that persisted beyond the expression of exogenous protein [38]. Finally, antibodies to TGFβ have been shown to attenuate bleomycin-induced pulmonary fibrosis in rats [39].

A number of other fibroblast mitogens have been implicated in pulmonary fibrosis both *in vitro* and *in vivo*. For example platelet derived growth factor (PDGF) and endothelin-1, in addition to their mitogenic action, are also fibroblast chemoattractants [40, 41]. This apparent plethora of fibroblast growth factors could represent a degree of redundancy in the repair system but it is equally possible that each factor will be of particular importance in a specific disease setting or at different stages of a disease process. We currently need to develop techniques to monitor growth factor activity within tissues and to assess the interaction between these factors within the complex extracellular environment.

4   The ying and the yang.

Attention has largely been focused on factors that promote collagen deposition in the lung. However, it is more likely that the progression to established fibrosis relies on a number of factors controlling the balance between matrix synthesis and degradation rates. Less is known about the role of these potentially inhibitory pathways. For example, Interferon gamma secreted by alveolar macrophages, inhibits fibroblast collagen synthesis *in vitro* [9, 42] and attenuates bleomycin-induced lung fibrosis when administered to mice [43].

Prostaglandin E_2 (PGE$_2$) is another potentially inhibitory cytokine. PGE$_2$ concentrations are decreased in broncho-alveolar lavage fluid form patients with idiopathic pulmonary fibrosis. In addition, fibroblasts from these patients demonstrate an enhanced response to TGF-β resulting from an impaired capacity to synthesise PGE$_2$ [44]. It has also been demonstrated in other tissues that PGE$_2$ inhibits the response of mesenchymal cells to other profibrotic cytokines such as angiotensin II [45].

Matrix components are susceptible to degradation by via a number of intracellular and extracellular pathways. The matrix metalloproteinases (MMP) capable of digesting collagens such as MMP-2 and MMP-9 [46] are elevated in the lungs of patients with ARDS but their relationship to the development of fibrosis or other outcomes is not known. For example, an elevation of the tissue inhibitors of metalloproteases (TIMPS) or an imbalance between these and their respective MMP's could lead to a more severe fibrotic response in some ARDS patients.

Finally, agents governing apoptotic rates amongst inflammatory and mesenchymal cells could result in a failure to clear these cells from sites of injury and lead to a persistence of the fibrotic process [47].

5 Profibrotic cytokines in ARDS.

Despite clinical and experimental evidence implicating a number of cytokines in the pathogenesis of chronic fibrotic lung disease over the past 20 years, they have received little attention in the context of ARDS [48]. This is perhaps surprising, given that animal models with the pathological and temporal features of acute lung injury rather than chronic fibrosis have been used to establish a number of these factors. TGFα is elevated in the oedema fluid of ARDS patients [49] and correlated with N-terminal procollagen peptide-III, a marker of collagen turnover [50]. Little is know about the physiological role of TGF-alpha however it is a potential fibroblast mitogen [51] A PDGF-like peptide which is chemotactic and mitogenic for fibroblasts has been also detected in ARDS BALF but it's contribution to the fibrotic process has not been established [52]. Moreover, clinical studies examining the role of other important profibrotic mediators such as TGFβ, endothelin-1, PDGF, insulin-like growth factor and basic fibroblast growth factor, implicated in chronic fibrotic disorders are lacking. There is likely to be overlap between the various interstitial lung diseases and these mediators warrant further attention.

6 Other profibrotic factors in ARDS.

Excessive mechanical forces generated during mechanical ventilation could contribute to the perpetuation of lung injury but have received little attention. Evidence suggests abnormal shear forces are generated between lung units of differing compliance and at the epithelial/endothelial interface, particularly when high pressure/volume ventilation strategies are employed [53, 54]. This leads to the exposure of damaged basement membranes -with implications for inflammatory and mesenchymal cell migration- and further vascular leakage. Experimentally, maintaining high pressure or high volume ventilation in animal models results in an acute lung injury syndrome resembling ARDS [55]. Furthermore, mechanical forces can directly stimulate matrix synthesis by a number of cell types *in vitro* [56] but their importance in lung injury has not been studied. High oxygen tensions themselves, comparable to those used in the treatment of ARDS and given for short periods of time can also induce lung injury experimentally, possibly via the generation of reactive oxidant species [57].

Such observations make an exacerbation of lung injury by mechanical ventilation likely. In an attempt to try and avoid these problems, lung-protective ventilation regimes aimed at reducing volutrauma and barotrauma whilst tolerating hypercapnoea and lower oxygen tensions are currently in use. In the future, perflurocarbon based liquid ventilation and high frequency oscillatory ventilation could, in theory, limit such forces in the lung, but we currently lack confirmation of clinical efficacy.

7 Fibroproliferation in ARDS when does it begin?

The classical descriptions of ARDS suggest that the initial exudative phase is followed by a proliferative and then a fibrotic phase[58]. These descriptions rest upon a number of histological studies which suffer from several problems, including clear identification of the onset of ARDS, the presence of a number of confounding variables including presence of nosocomial pneumonia, ventilator induced injury, concurrent use of steroids. In addition potential differences arise from different aetiological causes of ARDS and are exacerbated by the relative paucity of samples, most of which are post mortem. For these and other reasons the American-European consensus conference admitted that despite considerable effort they could not define the sequence of events leading to the pathological findings of ARDS [59]. This lack of understanding of the basic pathogenic mechanisms leading to pulmonary fibrosis has hampered progress towards effective therapeutic strategies. A fundamental aspect of the fibrosis seen in ARDS is that, unlike other pulmonary fibrotic conditions, it can resolve. Understanding how this resolution occurs would be a major advance.

Part of the difficulties in studying pulmonary fibrosis is in determining its onset and progression. Histological examination is the gold standard but lung biopsies are not commonly performed in ALI. Compliance measurements are relatively insensitive and not specific. Radiology is the mainstay for clinical evaluation but even CT is not specific, is difficult to quantify and to undertake repeated measurements. Another approach is to look at biochemical markers of collagen turnover such as the C and N-terminal peptides of procollagen I and III. N-terminal procollagen peptide (N-PCP-III) is one such marker and a trans-pulmonary gradient exists for this in normal lungs showing that collagen III is actively synthesised in the normal state [60]. Furthermore N-PCP-III has been shown to be elevated both in the serum and bronchoalveolar lavage of patients with ARDS [61]. Indeed recent studies demonstrate elevated N-PCP-III levels with 24 hours of mechanical ventilation for ARDS [50, 62]. Other recent studies also suggest that fibrosis may not simply be a late event as there is evidence of early increases in procollagen-I peptide levels and of myofibroblast cell numbers in alveolar walls in patients with ARDS [19]. Furthermore increased levels of N-PCP-III within 24 hours of ARDS are predictive of outcome with levels of over 1.75U/mlincreasing the risk of death more than four fold. Our studies have confirm that N-PCP-III is elevated within 48 hours in ARDS patients and that this can be detected in both BAL and serum [63]. This increase is specific to ARDS as N-PCP-III levels were not elevated in patients mechanically ventilated for cardiogenic pulmonary oedema who had a similar illness severity score and outcome to the ARDS cohort. Another key finding in this study was that the BAL fluid lavaged from ARDS patients within 48 hours of diagnosis was intensely mitogenic for fibroblasts. This all suggests that the fibrosis so characteristic of ARDS may not be a late event but is switched on at a remarkably early stage of the syndrome.

This may have implications for therapy. The only therapy of proven benefit for late ARDS with established fibrosis are steroids [64]. Three major trials of steroids in early ARDS demonstrated that they did not prevent the development of ARDS and that they increased the mortality [65 - 67]. Meduri however has shown that steroids have a place in late ARDS as a rescue therapy and significantly improved the outcome of patients with evidence of fibroproliferation. The exact timing of therapies to best prevent fibrosis while improving mortality now need to be established.

8   Conclusions.

ARDS is a clinical diagnosis and a heterogeneous group of patients are almost certainly encompassed by this term. Despite the difficulty in clinically defining ARDS, the majority of patients given this diagnosis appear to behave similarly in terms of their pathophysiological features, therapeutic requirements, clinical course and outcome. This undoubtedly reflects the involvement of common biological processes. Ultimately a better understanding of such events could lead to a improved profiling of patients and a more precise targeting of therapies to suit individuals. Thus, as our understanding of the pathogenic mechanisms improves, it may be more helpful in some ways, to consider a patient with ARDS as a combination of these responses to injury rather than a mixture of clinical signs and symptoms.

Anti-cytokine therapy will undoubtedly have an important place in our future therapeutic armoury and the identification of the key fibrotic factors involved in ARDS is an important goal. More sensitive and rapid techniques to monitor the fibrotic process and the efficacy of any new therapies will also need to occur in parallel and the procollagen peptides look particularly promising. Ultimately, it is likely that no single anti-fibrotic agent will be completely successful in ARDS given the complexity of the repair response and combination therapy is more likely. Thus it is important that we assess such therapies in terms of their ability to influence the fibrotic process and not just their effect on major outcomes such as mortality. There are currently a number of agents in development and we should be hopeful that they will become part of the future therapy for ARDS.

References.

1.   Hyers, T.M. and A.A. Fowler. (1986). Adult respiratory distress syndrome: causes, morbidity, and mortality. *Fed.Proc.* **45**:25-29.
2.   Suchyta, M.R., T.P. Clemmer, C.G. Elliott, J.F. Orme, and L.K. Weaver. (1992). The adult respiratory distress syndrome. A report of survival and modifying factors. *Chest* **101**:1074-1079.
3.   Raghu, G., L.J. Striker, L.D. Hudson, and G.E. Striker. (1985). Extracellular matrix in normal and fibrotic human lungs. *Am. Rev. Respir. Dis.* **131**:281-289.
4.   Zapol, W.M., R.L. Trelstad, J.W. Coffey, I. Tsai, and R.A. Salvador. (1979). Pulmonary fibrosis in severe acute respiratory failure. *Am. J. Respir. Crit. Care Med.* **119**:547-554.
5.   Montgomery, A.B., M.A. Stager, C.J. Carrico, and L.D. Hudson. (1985). Causes of mortality in patients with the adult respiratory distress syndrome. *Am. J. Respir. Crit. Care Med.* **132**:485-489.
6.   Bell, R.C., J.J. Coalson, J.D. Smith, and W.G. Johanson, Jr. (1983). Multiple organ system failure and infection in adult respiratory distress syndrome. *Ann. Intern. Med.* **99**:293-298.
7.   Donnelly, S.C., C. Haslett, I. Dransfield, C.E. Robertson, D.C. Carter, J.A. Ross, I.S. Grant, and T.F. Tedder. (1994). Role of selectins in development of adult respiratory distress syndrome [see comments]. *Lancet* **344**:215-219.
8.   Meduri, G.U., G. Kohler, S. Headley, E. Tolley, F. Stentz, and A. Postlethwaite. 1995. Inflammatory cytokines in the BAL of patients with ARDS. Persistent elevation over time predicts poor outcome. *Chest* **108**:1303-1314.
9.   Elias, J.A., B. Freundlich, S. Adams, and J. Rosenbloom. (1990). Regulation of human lung fibroblast collagen production by recombinant interleukin-1, tumor necrosis factor, and interferon-gamma. *Ann. N.Y. Acad. Sci.* **580**:233-44:233-244.
10.   Ortiz, L.A., J. Lasky, R.F. Hamilton, Jr., A. Holian, G.W. Hoyle, W. Banks, J.J. Peschon, A.R. Brody, G. Lungarella, and M. Friedman. (1998). Expression of TNF and the necessity of TNF receptors in bleomycin- induced lung injury in mice. *Exp. Lung Res.* **24**:721-743.
11.   Sueoka, N., E. Sueoka, Y. Miyazaki, S. Okabe, M. Kurosumi, S. Takayama, and H. Fujiki. 1998. Molecular pathogenesis of interstitial pneumonitis with TNF- alpha transgenic mice. *Cytokine.* **10**:124-131.
12.   Rom, W.N., P. Basset, G.A. Fells, T. Nukiwa, B.C. Trapnell, and R.G. Crysal. (1988). Alveolar macrophages release an insulin-like growth factor I- type molecule. *J. Clin. Invest.* **82**:1685-1693.
13.   Goldstein, R.H., C.F. Poliks, P.F. Pilch, B.D. Smith, and A. Fine. (1989). Stimulation of collagen formation by insulin and insulin-like growth factor-1 in cultures of human lung fibroblasts. *Endocrinology* **124**:964-970.
14.   Harrison, N.K., A.D. Cambrey, A.R. Myers, A.M. Southcott, C.M. Black, R.M. du Bois, G.J. Laurent, and R.J. McAnulty. (1994). Insulin-like growth factor-I is partially responsible for fibroblast proliferation induced by bronchoalveolar lavage fluid from patients with systemic sclerosis. *Clin. Sci.(Colch).* **86**:141-148.
15.   Henke, C., W. Marineili, J. Jessurun, J. Fox, D. Harms, M. Peterson, L. Chiang, and P. Doran. (1993). Macrophage production of basic fibroblast growth factor in the fibroproliferative disorder of alveolar fibrosis after lung injury. *Am. J. Pathol.* **143**:1189-1199.
16.   Donnelly, S.C., C. Haslett, P.T. Reid, I.S. Grant, W.A. Wallace, C.N. Metz, L.J. Bruce, and R. Bucala. (1997). Regulatory role for macrophage migration inhibitory factor in acute respiratory distress syndrome. *Nat. Med.* **3**:320-323.
17.   Armstrong, L. and A.B. Millar. (1997). Relative production of tumour necrosis factor alpha and interleukin 10 in adult respiratory distress syndrome. *Thorax* 52:442-446.

18. Weiland, J.E., W.B. Davis, J.F. Holter, J.R. Mohammed, P.M. Dorinsky, and J.E. Gadek. (1986). Lung neutrophils in the adult respiratory distress syndrome. Clinical and pathophysiologic significance. *Am. Rev. Respir. Dis.* **133**:218-225.

19. Liebler, J.M., Z. Qu, B. Buckner, M.R. Powers, and J.T. Rosenbaum. (1998). Fibroproliferation and mast cells in the acute respiratory distress syndrome. *Thorax* **53**:823-829.

20. Ruoss, S.J., T. Hartmann, and G.H. Caughey. (1991). Mast cell tryptase is a mitogen for cultured fibroblasts. *J. Clin. Invest.* **88**:493-499.

21. Sugahara, K., K. Iyama, M.J. Kuroda, and K. Sano. (1998). Double intratracheal instillation of keratinocyte growth factor prevents bleomycin-induced lung fibrosis in rats. *J Pathol.* **186**:90-98.

22. Deterding, R.R., A.M. Havill, T. Yano, S.C. Middleton, C.R. Jacoby, J.M. Shannon, W.S. Simonet, and R.J. Mason. (1997). Prevention of bleomycin-induced lung injury in rats by keratinocyte growth factor. *Proc. Assoc. Am. Physicians.* **109**:254-268.

23. Verghese GM, McCormick-Shannon K, Mason RJ, Matthay MA (1998) Hepatocyte growth factor and keratinocyte growth factor in the pulmonary edema fluid of patients with acute lung injury. Biologic and clinical significance. *Am. J. Respir. Crit. Care Med.* **158**: 386-94

24. Cambrey, A.D., O.J. Kwon, A.J. Gray, N.K. Harrison, M. Yacoub, P.J. Barnes, G.J. Laurent, and K.F. Chung. (1995). Insulin-like growth factor I is a major fibroblast mitogen produced by primary cultures of human airway epithelial cells. *Clin. Sci.(Colch).* **89**:611-617.

25. Adler, K.B., L.M. Callahan, and J.N. Evans. (1986). Cellular alterations in the alveolar wall in bleomycin-induced pulmonary fibrosis in rats. An ultrastructural morphometric study. *Am. Rev. Respir. Dis.* **133**:1043-1048.

26. Roberts, A.B., M.B. Sporn, R.K. Assoian, J.M. Smith, N.S. Roche, L.M. Wakefield, U.I. Heine, L.A. Liotta, V. Falanga, and J.H. Kehrl. (1986). Transforming growth factor type beta: rapid induction of fibrosis and angiogenesis in vivo and stimulation of collagen formation in vitro. *Proc. Natl. Acad. Sci. U.S.A.* **83**:4167-4171.

27. Ignotz, R.A. and J. Massague. (1986). Transforming growth factor beta stimulates the expression of fibronectin and collagen and their incorporation into the extracellular matrix. *J. Biol. Chem.* **261**:4337-4345.

28. Varga, J. and S.A. Jiminez. (1986). Stimulation of normal human fibroblast procollagen production and processing by transforming growth factor beta. *Biochem. Biophys. Acta.* **138**:974-980.

29. Raghow, R., A.E. Postlethwaite, J. Keski-Oja, H.L. Moses, and A.H. Kang. (1987). Transforming growth factor beta increases steady state levels of type I procollagen and fibronectin messenger mRNAs post-transcriptionally in cultured human dermal fibroblasts. *J. Clin. Invest.* **79**:1285-1288.

30. Ignotz, R.A., T. Endo, and J. Massague. (1987). Regulation of fibronectin and type I collagen mRNA levels by transforming growth factor-beta. *J. Biol. Chem.* **262**:6443-6446.

31. Edwards, D.R., G. Murphy, J.J. Reynolds, S.E. Whitham, A.J. Docherty, P. Angel, and J.K. Heath. (1987). Transforming growth factor beta modulates the expression of collagenase and metalloproteinase inhibitor. *EMBO J.* **6**:1899-1904.

32. Overall, C.M., J.L. Wrana, and J. Sodek. (1989). Independent regulation of collagenase, 72-kDa progelatinase, and metalloendoproteinase inhibitor expression in human fibroblasts by transforming growth factor-beta. *J. Biol. Chem.* **264**:1860-1869.

33. Hoyt, D.G. and J.S. Lazo. (1988). Alterations in pulmonary mRNA encoding procollagens, fibronectin and transforming growth factor-beta precede bleomycin-induced pulmonary fibrosis in mice. *J. Pharmacol. Exp. Ther.* **246**:765-771.

34. Hoyt, D.G. and J.S. Lazo. (1989). Early increases in pulmonary mRNA encoding procollagens and transforming growth factor-beta in mice sensitive to cyclophosphamide- induced pulmonary fibrosis. *J. Pharmacol. Exp. Ther.* **249**:38-43.

35. Broekelmann, T.J., A.H. Limper, T.V. Colby, and J.A. McDonald. (1991). Transforming growth factor beta 1 is present at sites of extracellular matrix gene expression in human pulmonary fibrosis. *Proc. Natl. Acad. Sci. U.S.A.* **88**:6642-6646.

36. Khalil, N., O. Bereznay, M. Sporn, and A.H. Greenberg. (1989). Macrophage production of transforming growth factor beta and fibroblast collagen synthesis in chronic pulmonary inflammation. *J. Exp. Med.* **170**:727-737.

37. McAnulty, R.J., N.A. Hernandez-Rodriguez, S.E. Mutsaers, R.K. Coker, and G.J. Laurent. (1997). Indomethacin suppresses the anti-proliferative effects of transforming growth factor-beta isoforms on fibroblast cell cultures. *Biochem. J.* **321**:639-643.

38. Sime, P.J., Z. Xing, F.L. Graham, K.G. Csaky, and J. Gauldie. (1997). Adenovector-mediated gene transfer of active transforming growth factor- beta1 induces prolonged severe fibrosis in rat lung. *J. Clin. Invest.* **100**:768-776.

39. Giri, S.N., D.M. Hyde, and M.A. Hollinger. (1993). Effect of antibody to transforming growth factor beta on bleomycin induced accumulation of lung collagen in mice [see comments]. *Thorax* **48**:959-966.

40.   Seppa, H., G. Grotendorst, S. Seppa, E. Schiffmann, and G.R. Martin. (1982). Platelet-derived growth factor in chemotactic for fibroblasts. *J Cell Biol.* 92:584-588.

41.   Peacock, A.J., K.E. Dawes, A. Shock, A.J. Gray, J.T. Reeves, and G.J. Laurent. (1992). Endothelin-1 and endothelin-3 induce chemotaxis and replication of pulmonary artery fibroblasts. *Am. J. Respir. Cell Moll. Biol.* 7:492-499.

42.   Clark, J.G., T.F. Dedon, E.A. Wayner, and W.G. Carter. (1989). Effects of interferon-gamma on expression of cell surface receptors for collagen and deposition of newly synthesized collagen by cultured human lung fibroblasts. *J. Clin. Invest.* 83:1505-1511.

43.   Gurujeyalakshmi, G. and S.N. Giri. (1995). Molecular mechanisms of antifibrotic effect of interferon gamma in bleomycin-mouse model of lung fibrosis: downregulation of TGF- beta and procollagen I and III gene expression. *Exp. Lung Res.* 21:791-808.

44.   Wilborn, J., L.J. Crofford, M.D. Burdick, S.L. .Kunkel, R.M. Streiter, and M. Peters-Golden. (1994). Cultured lung fibroblasts isolated from patients with idiopathic pulmonary fibrosis have a diminished capacity to synthesise prostaglandin E2 and to express cyclooxygenase-2. *J. Clin. Invest.* 95:1861-1868.

45.   Brilla, C.G., G. Zhou, H. Rupp, B. Maisch, and K.T. Weber. (1995). Role of angiotensin II and prostaglandin E2 in regulating cardiac fibroblast collagen turnover. *Am. J. Cardiol.* 76:8D-13D.

46.   Torii, K., K. Iida, Y. Miyazaki, S. Saga, Y. Kondoh, H. Taniguchi, F. Taki, K. Takagi, M. Matsuyama, and R. Suzuki. (1997). Higher concentrations of matrix metalloproteinases in bronchoalveolar lavage fluid of patients with adult respiratory distress syndrome. *Am. J. Respir. Crit. Care Med.* 155:43-46.

47.   Matute-Bello, G., W.C. Liles, F.2. Radella, K.P. Steinberg, J.T. Ruzinski, M. Jonas, E.Y. Chi, L.D. Hudson, and T.R. Martin. (1997). Neutrophil apoptosis in the acute respiratory distress syndrome. *Am. J. Respir. Crit. Care Med.* 156:1969-1977.

48.   McAnulty, R.J. and G.J. Laurent. (1995). Pathogenesis of lung fibrosis and potential new therapeutic strategies. *Exp. Nephrol.* 3:96-107.

49.   Madtes, D.K., G. Rubenfeld, L.D. Klima, J.A. Milberg, K.P. Steinberg, T.R. Martin, G. Raghu, L.D. Hudson, and J.G. Clark. (1998). Elevated transforming growth factor-alpha levels in bronchoalveolar lavage fluid of patients with acute respiratory distress syndrome. *Am. J. Respir. Crit. Care Med.* 158:424-430.

50.   Chesnutt, A.N., M.A. Matthay, F.A. Tibayan, and J.G. Clark. (1997). Early detection of type III procollagen peptide in acute lung injury. Pathogenic and prognostic significance. *Am. J. Respir. Crit. Care Med.* 156:840-845.

51.   Derynck, R., J.A. Jarrett, E.Y. Chen, and D.V. Goeddel. (1986). The murine transforming growth factor-beta precursor. *J. Biol. Chem.* 261:4377-4379.

52.   Snyder, L.S., M.I. Hertz, M.S. Peterson, K.R. Harmon, W.A. Marinelli, C.A. Henke, J.R. Greenheck, B. Chen, and P.B. Bitterman. (1991). Acute lung injury. Pathogenesis of intraalveolar fibrosis. *J. Clin. Invest.* 88:663-673.

53.   Parker, J.C., L.A. Hernandez, and K.J. Peevy. (1993). Mechanisms of ventilator-induced lung injury. *Crit. Care Med.* 21:131-143.

54.   Dreyfuss, D. and G. Saumon. (1993). Role of tidal volume, FRC, and end-inspiratory volume in the development of pulmonary edema following mechanical ventilation. *Am. Rev. Respir. Dis.* 148:1194-1203.

55.   Dreyfuss, D., P. Soler, G. Basset, and G. Saumon. (1988). High inflation pressure pulmonary edema. Respective effects of high airway pressure, high tidal volume, and positive end- expiratory pressure. *Am. Rev. Respir. Dis.* 137:1159-1164.

56.   Butt, R. and J.E. Bishop. (1997). Mechanical load enhances the stimulatory effect of serum growth factors on cardiac fibroblast collagen synthesis. *J. Moll. Cell Cardiol.* 29:1141-1151.

57.   Jackson, R.M. (1990). Molecular, pharmacologic, and clinical aspects of oxygen-induced lung injury. *Clin. Chest Med.* 11:73-86.

58.   Griffiths MJD and Evans TW (1995) Adult respiratory distress syndrome. *In* Respiratory Medicine (2nd Ed) Eds. Brewis RAL, Corrin, B Geddes DM and Gibson GJ. W.B. Saunders Press p605-629

59.   Bernard GR, Artigas A, Brigham KL, Carlet J, Falke K, Hudson L, Lamy M, Legall JR, Morris A, Spragg R (1994) The American-European Consensus Conference on ARDS. Definitions, mechanisms, relevant outcomes, and clinical trial co-ordination. *Am. J. Respir. Crit. Care Med.* 149: 818-24

60.   Harrison NK, Laurent GJ, Evans TW (1992) Transpulmonary gradient of type III procollagen peptides: acute effects of cardio-pulmonary bypass. Intensive Care Med 18; 290-292

61.   Entzian P, Huckstadt A, Kreipe H, Barth J (1990) Determination of serum concentrations of type III procollagen peptide in mechanically ventilated patients. Pronounced augmented concentrations in the adult respiratory distress syndrome. *Am. Rev. Respir. Dis.* 142; 1079-1082

62. Clark JG, Milberg JA, Steinberg KP, Hudson LD (1995) Type III procollagen peptide in the adult respiratory distress syndrome. Association of increased peptide levels in bronchoalveolar lavage fluid with increased risk for death *Ann. Intern. Med.* **122;** 17-23

63. R..P Marshall, G.J .Bellingan, A. Puddicome, N. Goldsack, R. Chambers, R. McAnulty, G.J. Laurent (1999) Early fibroproliferation in the acute respiratory distress syndrome. *Am. J. Respir. Crit. Care Med.* **159;** A378

64. Meduri GU, Headley AS, Golden E, Carson SJ, Umberger RA, Kelso T, Tolley EA (1998) Effect of prolonged methylprednisolone therapy in unresolving acute respiratory distress syndrome: a randomized controlled trial. *JAMA* **280;** 159-165

65. Luce JM, Montgomery AB, Marks JD, Turner J, Metz CA, Murray JF (1988) Ineffectiveness of high-dose methylprednisolone in preventing parenchymal lung injury and improving mortality in patients with septic shock. *Am. Rev. Respir. Dis.* **138;** 62-68

66. Bone RC, Fisher CJ Jr, Clemmer TP, Slotman GJ, Metz CA (1987) Early methylprednisolone treatment for septic syndrome and the adult respiratory distress syndrome. *Chest* **92;** 1032-1036

67. Bernard GR, Luce JM, Sprung CL, Rinaldo JE, Tate RM, Sibbald WJ, Kariman K, Higgins S, Bradley R, Metz CA, et al (1987) High-dose corticosteroids in patients with the adult respiratory distress syndrome. *N. Engl. J. Med.* **317;** 1565-1570.

Acute Lung Injury: From Inflammation to Repair
G.J. Bellingan and G.J. Laurent (Eds.)
IOS Press, 2000

Role of Thrombin in Lung Repair and Fibrosis

Rachel C. Chambers

Centre for Cardiopulmonary Biochemistry & Respiratory Medicine
Royal Free University College Medical School
Rayne Institute, London WC1E 6JJ, UK

1   Introduction.

Dramatic activation of the coagulation cascade is a frequent consequence of acute lung injury (ALI). This chapter will review the evidence that a number of products generated as a result of the activation of the coagulation cascade ALI play important roles in subsequent inflammatory and tissue repair processes, and thereby contribute to lung pathology in ALI and the acute respiratory distress syndrome (ARDS). The roles of fibrin(ogen) and fibrin(ogen) breakdown products in this regard are well recognized and have been extensively documented (for a review see [1]). This chapter will therefore only briefly review this literature and will focus on the final enzyme of the coagulation cascade, namely the serine protease, thrombin. This enzyme, besides its critical role in haemostasis, exerts a number of cellular effects, including promoting platelet aggregation, inflammatory cell trafficking, fibroblast proliferation and the induction of pro-inflammatory and pro-fibrotic cytokines and growth factors.

This chapter will begin with a detailed description of the coagulation cascade, since an understanding on how thrombin is generated and how its activity is regulated will be important for an understanding of its physiological functions and its potential role in normal lung repair, inflammation and fibrosis. This will be followed by a description of the evidence that the coagulation cascade is abnormally activated in the lungs of patients with ALI/ARDS. The final sections will discuss the mechanism by which products of the coagulation cascade may contribute to lung pathology, with a particular focus on the cellular effects of thrombin and its potential role in promoting inflammation and lung fibrosis.

2   The coagulation cascade.

2.1   Activation of the coagulation cascade.

The coagulation cascade is usually only initiated upon tissue injury involving damage to the vasculature. It main function is to ensure the formation of a stable haemostatic clot to plug injured vessels and prevent further blood loss. The provisional clot comprises aggregated platelets enmeshed by insoluble fibrin, as a result of the action of thrombin, the final enzyme generated as a result of the stepwise activation of serine proteases via two highly regulated pathways, termed the extrinsic and intrinsic coagulation systems (for a schematic diagram of the coagulation cascade, see Figure 1 and for further details refer to [2]).

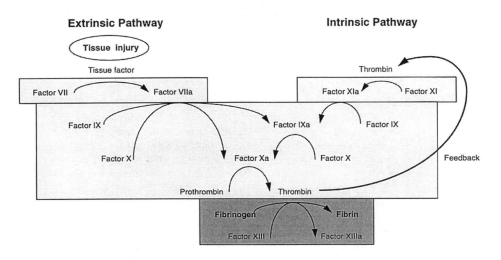

Figure 1. The Coagulation Cascade. The coagulation cascade involves the stepwise activation of serine proteases via the extrinsic and intrinsic pathways. At the point of convergence of these two pathways, factor Xa converts inactive prothrombin to active thrombin. Thrombin in turn acts upon soluble fibrinogen to form insoluble fibrin.

The **extrinsic pathway** is usually initiated when tissue factor, expressed on the surface of activated vascular endothelial cells and platelets following damage to blood vessels, binds circulating factor VII which in turn is activated and forms the proteinase complex in association with cell surface phospholipids and calcium ions (Ca^{2+}). The main function of this complex is to activate factor X, as well as limited amounts of factor IX.

The alternative activation pathway, or **intrinsic pathway** is triggered when blood comes into contact with negatively-charged components of the subendothelial connective tissue, such as collagen. This pathway is initiated by the kallikrein-kinin system and results in the sequential activation of factors XII, XI and IX, although it can also be triggered by a range of cell types, including monocytes and alveolar macrophages. Factor IXa, in association with factor VIIIa, phospholipids and Ca^{2+}, activates factor X at the point of convergence of the two coagulation pathways. Activated factor X in turn binds to a newly described integral cell surface receptor, termed effector protease receptor-1 (EPR-1) on the surface of a number of cell types, including platelets, inflammatory cells and endothelial cells ([3] and references therein). Factor Xa bound to EPR-1, in association with factor Va, phospholipids and Ca^{2+} forms the prothrombinase complex, responsible for the conversion of prothrombin to thrombin. Thrombin finally cleaves the soluble plasma protein fibrinogen to insoluble fibrin, and activates factor XIII, which in turn crosslinks and stabilizes the nascent fibrin clot. At the same time, thrombin also promotes platelet aggregation and degranulation with the resultant formation of stable haemostatic plugs.

In terms of the respective roles of the two coagulation pathways, it has been proposed that the **extrinsic pathway** serves to initiate blood coagulation and generate limited amounts of factor Xa and thrombin. These then feed back into the **intrinsic coagulation** pathway which is ultimately responsible for the dramatic amplification of the initial signal and the generation of physiologically relevant concentrations of thrombin and sustained blood coagulation [2].

2.2   Activation of the coagulation cascade independent of blood coagulation.

The coagulation cascade can also be activated independently of blood coagulation. For example, a number of cells, including macrophages, fibroblasts, epithelial cells and smooth muscle cells express tissue factor [4] and are therefore capable of triggering the extrinsic coagulation cascade. Although tissue factor expression in the normal lung is very low, its expression has been shown to be dramatically increased in the inflamed and fibrotic lung, where it is predominantly associated with alveolar macrophages, as well as type II pneumocytes in close association with fibrin deposits [5]. Inflammatory cells such as monocytes and neutrophils express EPR-1 and therefore also support the formation of the prothrombinase complex [6]. More recently, certain viruses and bacterial proteases have been reported to promote the generation of factor Xa and are therefore capable of triggering the full activation of the coagulation cascade [7]. Finally, increased microvascular permeability alone can promote tissue fibrin deposition. Since increased microvascular permeability is a characteristic feature of ARDS [8], it may be a major contributor to extravascular coagulation and fibrin deposition in the lungs of patients with this condition.

2.3   Switching-off the coagulation cascade.

In normal non-disease states, blood coagulation is tightly controlled by both negative feedback mechanisms, as well as by circulating and locally-produced inhibitors. The major protease inhibitor responsible for the early shut-down of the extrinsic pathway is a protein termed tissue factor pathway inhibitor (TFPI). This protein inactivates factor Xa and forms an inactive binary complex which combines with factor VIIa/tissue factor. The intrinsic pathway is mainly controlled by antithrombin III which inhibits thrombin and other serine proteases of the coagulation cascade in the presence of heparin. Other important physiological inhibitors include, heparin cofactor II and protease nexin-1 which inhibit thrombin, and α_2-macroglobulin and α_1-antitrypsin (also known as α_1-proteinase inhibitor) which have a broader substrate specificity and inhibit thrombin, factor IXa, Xa and XIa (reviewed in [2]). Finally, blood coagulation is also regulated when thrombin binds to an endothelial cell surface receptor, termed thrombomodulin, and is converted from a procoagulant to an anticoagulant by activating protein C. Protein C, in conjunction with its cofactor protein S, inactivates factors Va and VIIIa and thereby prevents further thrombin generation.

3   The coagulation cascade in ALI/ARDS.

3.1   Evidence for excessive and persistent activation of the coagulation cascade.

Dramatic activation of the coagulation cascade has been extensively documented for both adults and newborn infants with ALI. Indeed, extensive fibrin deposition in interstitial and intraalveolar spaces, where it is a major component of hyaline membranes, is a characteristic feature of ALI/ARDS (reviewed in [1]). There is also evidence for intravascular coagulation, in the form of fibrin deposits and pulmonary microemboli within intravascular compartments [9]. Consistent with these findings, studies on bronchoalveolar lavage fluid (BALF) obtained from patients with ALI/ARDS have demonstrated that this fluid contains increased procoagulant activity, as well as procoagulant markers in the form of thrombin-antithrombin complexes (TAT complexes), prothrombin fragment 1.2 and fibrin fragments ([10] and references therein). However, although its presence is clearly implied by the deposition of fibrin, it has not been possible to detect active thrombin directly in bronchoalveolar lavage fluid from patients with ARDS. Indeed, most of the detectable procoagulant activity present in bronchoalveolar lavage fluid was shown to be attributable to tissue factor-factor VII/VIIa complexes, which are capable of initiating coagulation by activating factor X [11]. In terms of the cells responsible for generating tissue factor procoagulant activity within the alveolar compartment, current evidence points towards the alveolar macrophage, although as discussed above, there is also increasing evidence that other lung cells, including epithelial cells, lung fibroblasts and type II pneumocytes may contribute to procoagulant responses of the injured lung [5]. In addition to tissue-factor procoagulant activity, there is also evidence for a small amount of prothrombinase-like activity in BALF from patients with ARDS [11]. These findings in patients are supported by studies in various animal models of ALI/ARDS, such as those induced following intratracheal instillation of oleic acid or bleomycin [1].

In addition to evidence for excessive activation of the coagulation cascade, there are also reports that the persistence of fibrin deposits and hyaline membranes in the lungs of patients with ALI/ARDS may be due to reduced thrombin inhibition and abnormal fibrinolysis. For example, levels of a number of circulating endogenous anticoagulants, including antithrombin III, protein C and protein S have been shown to be reduced in these patients [12]. Evidence for increased antifibrinolytic activity in the bronchoalveolar compartment of patients with ARDS has also been reported [13]. This includes increased levels of urokinase inhibitors, such as plasminogen activator inhibitor (PAI-1), as well as increased antiplasmin activity.

3.2   Role of the coagulation cascade in pulmonary fibrosis.

There is a wealth of evidence suggesting that activation of the coagulation cascade, with persistent fibrin deposition, contributes to the pathogenesis of acute lung. A number of these products have been shown to increase endothelial permeability, exacerbate pulmonary hypertension and amplify lung inflammation and inactivate surfactant ([14] and references therein). It is also very likely that a number of these products may play an important role in promoting pulmonary fibrosis following acute lung injury.

Excessive and abnormal deposition of interstitial collagens is common consequence of acute lung injury. Indeed extensive interstitial and intra-alveolar fibrosis are hallmarks of the more advanced stages of ARDS, although there is now increasing evidence that lung collagen turnover is increased at the very earliest stages in ARDS [15,16]. The fibrotic response following ALI/ARDS is indistinguishable from that which occurs in more chronic forms of interstitial lung disease, such as cryptogenic fibrosing alveolitis (CFA, also known as idiopathic pulmonary fibrosis or IPF) [17]. The current most favoured hypothesis for the pathogenesis of pulmonary fibrosis proposes that injury to the lung leads to inflammation and infiltration of inflammatory cells, including neutrophils, macrophages and lymphocytes. These, together with activated resident lung cells, are then thought to release a host of mediators, including cytokines and growth factors, which in turn stimulate local fibroblasts to migrate to sites of injury, replicate and produce excessive connective tissue proteins. However, little is known about the mediators involved in driving fibroproliferation and fibrogenesis in ALI/ARDS.

In addition to classical growth factors and cytokines, there is increasing evidence that products of the coagulation cascade may play an important role in driving the fibrotic response. Fibrin deposition and increased tissue factor expression are also common features in the lungs of patients with chronic forms of pulmonary fibrosis, including patients with CFA and pulmonary fibrosis associated with systemic sclerosis (SSc) [5,18]. Consistent with these findings, we and others have also shown that thrombin levels are increased in the lungs of patients with pulmonary fibrosis associated with SSc [19,20]. Further support for a role for the coagulation cascade in pulmonary fibrosis comes from studies in animal models of pulmonary fibrosis following ALI in which thrombin levels, tissue factor expression and fibrin deposition have also been shown to be increased [21].

4   Role of fibrin(ogen) in lung repair and fibrosis.

Early studies on the role of coagulation cascade in ALI/ARDS focused on the role of fibrin(ogen) and fibrin(ogen) degradation products. It is now clear that fibrin turnover extends beyond traditional haemostasis and plays a pivotal role in influencing subsequent inflammatory responses and tissue repair mechanisms. As well as providing a provisional structural matrix for fibroblasts and inflammatory cells migrating into the area of injury, fibrin also binds a number of mediators, including transforming growth factor-β (TGFβ) and platelet-derived growth factor (PDGF), and therefore acts as a reservoir of growth factors and fibrogenic cytokines [22]. There is also *in vitro* evidence that various fibrin(ogen) degradation products, including the Aα and Bβ chains of fibrin(ogen), as well as the fibrinopeptides A and B generated by thrombin cleavage, can act as mitogens for human lung fibroblasts [23] and influence the recruitment of inflammatory cells [24]; whereas certain fibrin degradation products have been shown to affect vascular permeability and promote lung inflammation *in vivo* [25]. Furthermore, studies in transgenic mice either lacking or overexpressing the murine PAI-1 gene showed that alterations in fibrinolytic activity had a strong influence on the extent of pulmonary fibrosis induced following intratracheal instillation of bleomycin [26]. Given the widespread deposition and persistence of fibrin in the lungs of patients with ALI/ARDS, it is therefore highly likely that fibrin(ogen) and fibrin degradation products play important roles in promoting lung inflammation and influencing the deposition of excessive matrix proteins in the lungs of these patients.

5   Role of thrombin in lung repair and fibrosis.

In terms of influencing inflammation and tissue repair processes thrombin has received the lion's share of attention amongst all proteases of the coagulation cascade. Indeed, intense research efforts over the last fifteen years has led to the realization that thrombin exerts multiple effects on a wide variety of cells and besides influencing platelet aggregation, also promotes the migration of inflammatory cells and the proliferation of mesenchymal cells. There is some evidence that thrombin, when bound to the subendothelial matrix, is protected from inactivation by antiproteases and can therefore remain functional and available for cellular interactions [27], so that it's cellular effects may persist beyond blood coagulation. Most of thrombin's cellular effects are not mediated directly by thrombin but rather via the induction and release of secondary mediators. A number of these may be part of the normal response to tissue injury, but in states where there is excessive and/or persistent activation of the coagulation cascade, it is likely that thrombin may contribute to lung pathology via both its procoagulant and cellular effects (for summary, please see Figure 2). The remaining discussion of this chapter will focus on the role of thrombin in inflammation, tissue repair and fibrosis, but readers are referred to excellent recent reviews for further details of all of thrombin's cellular effects in a variety of organs [28,29].

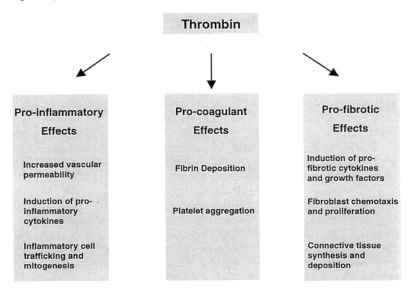

Figure 2. Putative role of thrombin in lung inflammation and fibrosis.

5.1   Thrombin receptors.

Most of thrombin's cellular effects are mediated via a number of ubiquitously expressed cell surface receptors called protease-activated receptors (PARs). At least four PARs have been characterized to date, but only three (PAR-1, -3 and -4) act as thrombin receptors [30, 31, 32]. The name of these receptors is derived from their unique mode of activation which involves limited proteolysis of specific amino acid sequences from their N-terminus rather than direct ligand binding [30] (for a diagrammatic representation please see Figure 3). This results in the generation of a new N-terminus which in turn functions as a tethered ligand and binds intramolecularly to body of the receptor and thereby induces a change in receptor conformation allowing the activated receptor to interact with heterotrimeric G proteins. These in turn initiate the formation of second messengers and cell signalling. Synthetic peptides corresponding to the tethered ligand of both PAR-1 and PAR-4 are capable of mimicking certain thrombin responses in cells expressing these receptors and are commonly used to invoke the involvement of these receptors in mediating a particular cellular effect influenced by thrombin. In contrast, synthetic peptides corresponding to the tethered ligand sequence of PAR-3 are not capable of activating this receptor.

Most of thrombin's cellular effects involved in tissue repair appear to be mediated via PAR-1, the first thrombin receptor to be cloned and characterized. PAR-1 has a wide tissue distribution and is present on most cells, including platelets, endothelial cells, epithelial cells, fibroblasts, smooth muscle cells, monocytes, lymphocytes, and certain tumor cell lines (reviewed in [29]). PAR-3 and PAR-4 gene transcripts have been detected in most human tissues examined, including the lung, but the expression of PAR-4 on platelets appears to be much lower than for PAR-1 [32]. The exact roles of these multiple thrombin receptors remains at present uncertain but given that thrombin activates them with different potency (high for PAR-1 and PAR-3; low for PAR-4), it has been suggested that the existence of multiple receptors may allow cells to respond to a wide range of thrombin concentrations in a graded manner. Finally, in addition to the three PARs, thrombin has also been reported to activate certain cell types, including smooth muscle cells, fibroblasts and endothelial cells via a non-proteolytic mechanism, but the nature of the receptor(s) involved remain(s) at present unknown.

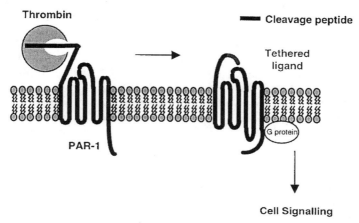

Figure 3. Model of activation of protease-activated receptors. Thrombin cleaves its receptors at their amino-terminus and unmasks a tethered ligand which interacts with the body of the receptor and induces conformational changes allowing it to interact with heterotrimeric G-proteins (modified from [30]).

5.2   Cellular effects of thrombin.

5.2.1   Platelet activation.

The earliest cellular response initiated by thrombin at sites of vascular injury, involves its interaction with platelets, which as a consequence of thrombin activation, aggregate and release thromboxane A2, platelet factor 4, as well as fibrogenic mediators involved in influencing early tissue repair responses, such as PDGF and TGFβ [33]. The effects of thrombin on human platelet aggregation can be mimicked with synthetic activating peptides for PAR-1 and can be blocked with PAR-1 neutralizing antibodies, indicating that PAR-1 plays a critical role in mediating the effects of thrombin on human platelets. In contrast, studies with PAR-1 and PAR-3 knockout mice revealed that PAR-1-deficient mouse platelets respond normally to thrombin [34] and that PAR-3 was responsible for mediating normal thrombin responses in mouse platelets [35]. The recent observation that PAR-4 activating peptides were shown to mimic the effects of thrombin on platelet secretion in mice has lead to the suggestion of the existence of a dual thrombin receptor system in the mouse, where platelet aggregation is predominantly mediated by PAR-3 and secretion is mediated by PAR-4 [35]. Although not yet conclusive, there is some evidence that a dual-receptor system involving PAR-1 and PAR-4 may also exist in humans.

5.2.2   Vascular tone and permeability.

In addition to influencing platelet function, thrombin exerts dramatic effects on vascular tone by an endothelial-dependent mechanism involving the release of nitric oxide and by directly causing the contraction of vascular smooth muscle (for a recent review please see [29]). Thrombin and PAR-1 activating peptides have also been shown to affect vascular permeability via both direct effects on endothelial cells [36], and via the release of serotonin from platelets and histamine from mast cells [37]. Increased vascular permeability is a characteristic feature of ALI/ARDS, and direct intravenous infusion of thrombin has been shown to increase pulmonary vascular permeability in experimental animals [38], but whether thrombin is playing a role via its direct cellular effects on the pulmonary vasculature in humans with ALI/ARDS remains at present uncertain.

5.2.3   Inflammatory cell trafficking.

Thrombin also exerts potent pro-inflammatory effects and may therefore play a key role during the inflammatory phase of ALI/ARDS. It is a potent chemoattractant for inflammatory cells ([39] and references therein) and stimulates the release of chemoattractants and pro-inflammatory cytokines, including monocyte chemotactic factor-1 (MCP-1), interleukin-6 (IL-6) and IL-8 by a number of cell types [40,41]. Thrombin further influences the trafficking of inflammatory cells by inducing the expression of endothelial cell surface adhesion molecules, such as P-selectin and intercellular adhesion molecule-1 (ICAM-1) [42]. The pivotal role of both the neutrophil and IL-8 in ALI/ARDS is well established and was elegantly demonstrated in a recent study in which a monoclonal antibody to IL-8 almost completely prevented pulmonary edema and alveolar destruction in an animal model of ARDS induced by endotoxaemia [43]. However, there is, to date, no *in vivo* evidence that thrombin contributes to the production of IL-8 or other inflammatory cytokines in ALI/ARDS directly.

5.2.4   Pro-fibrotic effects.

It has been known for several years, that thrombin may influence normal tissue repair processes as it is a potent mitogen for a variety of cell types, including fibroblasts, endothelial cells and smooth muscle cells [44, 45]. Considerable research efforts over the last ten years have indeed provided compelling evidence that thrombin plays a major role in the renewal of damaged blood vessels, as well as in a number of vascular pathologies associated with hyperproliferation of vascular smooth muscle cells, such as restenosis following vascular injury [46] and atherosclerosis [47]. The mitogenic and pro-fibrotic effects of thrombin will be considered in some detail in this chapter, since these effects may be particularly important during the "fibroproliferative phase" of ALI/ARDS, as well as in chronic interstitial lung disease associated with excessive and persistent activation of the coagulation cascade.

5.2.5   Fibroblast function.

In terms of influencing fibroblast proliferation, recent evidence from experiments employing PAR-1 activating peptides and fibroblasts derived from PAR-1 knockout mice suggests that PAR-1 is the predominant thrombin receptor involved [48]. As for a number of thrombin's cellular effects, thrombin does not promote fibroblast proliferation directly but rather via the induction and secretion of autocrine growth factors, including PDGF-AA and PDGF-AB [49]. In this regard, a thrombin response element was recently characterized in the PDGF B-chain gene promoter region in endothelial cells [50]. In addition to inducing PDGF-AA by cultured human lung fibroblasts, thrombin has also been shown to up-regulate PDGF α-receptor expression [20], ensuring that the target cell is capable of responding to the autocrine mediator induced. The mitogenic effects of thrombin may play an important role in expanding fibroblast numbers at sites of tissue injury and although there have, to date, been no studies on the role of thrombin as a fibroblast mitogen in ALI/ARDS, we have previously shown that thrombin was a major fibroblast mitogen present in bronchoalveolar lavage fluid obtained from patients with pulmonary fibrosis associated with SSc in in vitro proliferation studies [19]. In addition to being a mitogen, thrombin has also been shown to be a fibroblast chemoattractant [51] and may therefore also contribute to expanding fibroblasts at sites of injury by recruitment from neighbouring environments.

Thrombin also exerts stimulatory effects on connective tissue protein production by cultured mesenchymal cells. It is a potent promoter of fibronectin production and release by cultured fibroblasts and epithelial cells [52] and exerts both stimulatory and inhibitory effects on proteoglycan protein production in vitro [53]. More recently, we have shown that thrombin also increases procollagen production by human lung fibroblasts [54] and vascular smooth muscle cells [55]. We have further shown that these effects occur independently of changes in cell proliferation and are mediated, at least in part, via increased procollagen $\alpha_1(I)$ mRNA levels. The stimulatory effects of thrombin on procollagen production could further be mimicked with PAR-1 activating peptides, whereas fibroblasts from PAR-1-deficient mice appeared to be totally unresponsive, suggesting that these effects are mediated via activation of PAR-1. Finally, the stimulatory effects of thrombin on procollagen mRNA levels were delayed and could be abolished with cycloheximide, suggesting that thrombin again exerts its effects via a newly synthesized protein product rather than a direct mechanism. Current research in our laboratory is focused on elucidating the nature of this protein using oligonucleotide microarray technology which allows the simultaneous monitoring of changes in mRNA levels for thousands of genes on a single oligonucleotide microarray. Finally, in addition to its direct effects on procollagen synthesis, there is also in vitro evidence that thrombin promotes the basolateral secretion of pre-stored collagen by endothelial cells [56], increases collagen lattice contraction by fibroblasts [57] and promotes the production of activation of matrix metalloproteinases [58]. Taken together these observations support the concept that thrombin may also play a role in influencing the remodelling of the nascent matrix during tissue repair in vivo.

5.2.6   Tissue repair and fibrosis in vivo.

Support for the hypothesis that thrombin promotes connective tissue synthesis and deposition in vivo has come from studies in which thrombin and thrombin receptor agonists have been used to enhance wound healing responses and neovascularization in experimental animals [59]. However, studies performed with PAR-1-deficient mice have thus far failed to support a critical role for this receptor in the setting of skin wound healing responses [60]. Despite these findings, studies with direct thrombin inhibitors or PAR-1 blocking antibodies have provided compelling evidence that thrombin and PAR-1 are playing critical roles in a number of fibroproliferative disorders associated with hyperproliferation of smooth muscle cells and neointima formation following vascular injury [61,62].

Although there is good evidence that thrombin levels are increased in both animal models of acute lung injury [21] and in patients with pulmonary fibrosis [19,20], there are, to date, no published studies showing that thrombin contributes to pulmonary fibrosis directly. We have begun to address this question in an animal model of pulmonary fibrosis following acute lung injury induced by the intratracheal instillation of bleomycin, using a direct thrombin inhibitor (UK156406 generously made available to us by Pfizer, UK) delivered continuously via an osmotic minipump. In very encouraging preliminary experiments, we have been able to show that the typical doubling in lung collagen accumulation obtained 14 days after bleomycin administration can be blocked by up to 40% in animals receiving the direct thrombin inhibitor compared with animals receiving drug vehicle alone. Studies to determine whether the protective effects of the thrombin inhibitor are primarily due to blocking the cellular effects of thrombin (pro-inflammatory and pro-fibrotic) or via its haemostatic effects (i.e. deposition of intra- and extra-vascular fibrin) are still ongoing.

This is, to our knowledge, the first demonstration that thrombin may play an important role in promoting lung collagen accumulation in an *in vivo model* of ALI. However, in terms of adopting such an approach for use in patients with ALI/ARDS, there are serious concerns that direct thrombin inhibition may lead to bleeding complications, in particular since platelet counts and circulating antithrombin III levels are reduced in these patients. With the recent discovery of the existence of multiple thrombin receptors with tissue-specific roles, a number of pharmaceutical companies and academic groups have begun to develop novel therapeutic agents that will selectively block thrombin's different cellular actions without affecting its critical role in blood coagulation. In this regard, there have been considerable efforts to develop compounds primarily aimed at blocking PAR-1 as novel anti-thrombotic agents and for preventing restenosis following vascular injury (for a recent review see [63]). This includes PAR-1 antagonists and blocking antibodies designed to block PAR-1 activation, as well as PAR-1 antisense oligonucleotides to block PAR-1 mRNA translation and expression of the receptor at the cell surface. Studies with these agents in the context of pulmonary fibrosis should provide definitive evidence for the importance of thrombin-mediated cellular events in the pathogenesis of these disorders.

6.   Summary and conclusions.

There is a wealth of evidence to suggest that thrombin and other products of the coagulation cascade may play an important role in lung inflammation and fibrosis associated with ALI/ARDS. First, there is evidence for dramatic activation of the coagulation cascade in both patients and in animal models of this condition. Second, it is now well established that thrombin influences a number of subsequent inflammatory and tissue repair responses. Third, although, the exact pathophysiological role of the cellular effects of thrombin in pulmonary inflammation and fibrosis following acute lung injury in humans remains to be established, animal studies with direct thrombin inhibitors and genetically modified mice suggest that interfering with the coagulation cascade may be a beneficial approach to prevent excess collagen deposition following ALI. With the discovery that the cellular effects of thrombin are mediated via multiple receptors with tissue-specific roles and that both the pro-inflammatory and pro-fibrotic effects of thrombin appear to be predominantly mediated via PAR-1, this receptor may represent a novel target for preventing inflammation and pulmonary fibrosis associated with excessive activation and extravasation of serine proteases of the coagulation cascade. Strategies aimed at blocking this receptor may prove particularly beneficial since it has the advantage over direct thrombin inhibition in that it avoids the risk of provoking bleeding complications. The usefulness of PAR-1 antagonists as therapeutic agents for ALI/ARDS awaits confirmation but this information should be forthcoming as we continue to develop better agents and unravel the exact role of this receptor in the disease process.

Acknowledgements.

The author acknowledges generous support from The Wellcome Trust (Programme Grant No 051154) and the Medical Research Council for funding research on the role of thrombin in pulmonary fibrosis. The author also thanks Mr Olivier Blanc-Brude for preparing Figures 1 and 3.

References.

1.   S. Idell. (1994) Extravascular coagulation and fibrin deposition in acute lung injury, *New Horizons* **2** 566-574.
2.   E.W. Davie. (1995) Biochemical and molecular aspects of the coagulation cascade, *Thrombosis and Haemostasis* **74** 1-6.
3.   F. Bono, J.P. Herault, C. Avril, P. Schaeffer, J.C. Lormeau, J.M. Herbert. (1997) Human umbilical vein endothelial cells express high affinity receptors for factor Xa, *Journal of Cellular Physiology* 172 36-43.
4.   H.J. Brinkman, K. Mertens, J. Holthuis, L.A. Zwart-Huinink, K. Grijm, J.A. van Mourik. (1994) The activation of human blood coagulation factor X on the surface of endothelial cells: a comparison with various vascular cells, platelets and monocytes, *British Journal of Haematology* **87** 332-342.
5.   S. Imokawa, A. Sato, H. Hayakawa, M. Kotani, T. Urano, A. Takada. (1997) Tissue factor expression and fibrin deposition in the lungs of patients with idiopathic pulmonary fibrosis and systemic sclerosis, *American Journal of Respiratory and Critical Care Medicine* **156** 631-636.
6.   D.C. Altieri, T.S. Edgington. (1989) Sequential receptor cascade for coagulation proteins on monocytes. Constitutive biosynthesis and functional prothrombinase activity of a membrane form of factor V/Va, *Journal o Biological Chemistry* **264** 2969-2972.
7.   T. Imamura, J. Potempa, S. Tanase, J. Travis. (1997) Activation of blood coagulation factor X by arginine-specific cysteine proteinases (gingipain-Rs) from Porphyromonas gingivalis, *Journal of Biological Chemistry* **272** 16062-16067.
8.   H.F. Dvorak, S.J. Galli, A.M. Dvorak. (1986) Cellular and vascular manifestations of cell-mediated immunity, *Human Pathology* **17** 122-137.
9.   R.C. Bone, P.B. Francis, A.K. Pierce. (1976 Intravascular coagulation associated with the adult respiratory distress syndrome, *American Journal of Medicine* **61**) 585-589.
10.   J.T. Owings, R. Gosselin. (1997) Acquired antithrombin deficiency following severe traumatic injury: rationale for study of antithrombin supplementation, *Seminars in Thrombosis and Hemostasis* **23** Suppl 1 17-24.
11.   Idell S, Gonzalez K, and Bradford H. (1987) Procoagulant activity in bronchoalveolar lavage in the adult respiratory distress syndrome. Contribution of tissue factor associated with factor VII. *American Review of Respiratory Disease*;**136**: 1466-74.
12.   S.B. Sheth, A.C. Carvalho. (1991) Protein S and C alterations in acutely ill patients, *American Journal of Hematology* **36** 14-19.
13.   P. Bertozzi, B. Astedt, L. Zenzius, K. Lynch, F. LeMaire, W. Zapol, H.A. Chapman, Jr (1990). Depressed bronchoalveolar urokinase activity in patients with adult respiratory distress syndrome, *New England Journal of Medicine* **322** 890-897.
14.   K. Abubakar, B. Schmidt, S. Monkman, C. Webber, D. deSa, R. (1998) Roberts. Heparin improves gas exchange during experimental acute lung injury in newborn piglets, *American Journal of Respiratory and Critical Care Medicine* **158** 1620-1625.
15.   A.N. Chesnutt, M.A. Matthay, F.A. Tibayan, J.G. Clark. (1997) Early detection of type III procollagen peptide in acute lung injury. Pathogenetic and prognostic significance, *American Journal of Respiratory and Critical Care Medicine* **156** 840-845.
16.   G.U. Meduri, E.A. Tolley, A. Chinn, F. Stentz, A. Postlethwaite. (1998) Procollagen types I and III aminoterminal propeptide levels during acute respiratory distress syndrome and in response to methylprednisolone treatment, *American Journal of Respiratory and Critical Care Medicine* **158** 1432-1441.
17.   G. Raghu, L.J. Striker, L.D. Hudson, G.E. Striker. (1985) Extracellular matrix in normal and fibrotic human lungs, *American Review of Respiratory Disease* **131** 281-289.
18.   C. Kuhn, 3d, J. Boldt, T.E. King, Jr., E. Crouch, T. Vartio, J.A. McDonald. (1989) An immunohistochemical study of architectural remodelling and connective tissue synthesis in pulmonary fibrosis, *American Review of Respiratory Disease* **140** 1693-1703.

19.   N.A. Hernandez Rodriguez, A.D. Cambrey, N.K. Harrison, R.C. Chambers, A.J. Gray, A.M. Southcott, R.M. duBois, C.M. Black, M.F. Scully, R.J. McAnulty, et al. (1995) Role of thrombin in pulmonary fibrosis, Lancet 346 1071-1073.

20.   T. Ohba, J.K. McDonald, R.M. Silver, C. Strange, E.C. LeRoy, A. Ludwicka. (1994) Scleroderma bronchoalveolar lavage fluid contains thrombin, a mediator of human lung fibroblast proliferation via induction of platelet-derived growth factor alpha-receptor, American Journal of Respiratory Cell and Molecular Biology 10 405-412.

21.   K.S. Tani, F. Yasuoka, K. Ogushi, K. Asada, T. Fujisawa, T. Ozaki, N. Sano, T. Ogura. (1991) Thrombin enhances lung fibroblast proliferation in bleomycin-induced pulmonary fibrosis, American Journal of Respiratory Cell and Molecular Biology 5: 34-40.

22.   D.J. Grainger, L. Wakefield, H.W. Bethell, R.W. Farndale, J.C. Metcalfe. (1995) Release and activation of platelet latent TGF-beta in blood clots during dissolution with plasmin, Nature Medicine 1 932-937.

23.   A.J. Gray, J.E. Bishop, J.T. Reeves, G.J. Laurent. (1993)A alpha and B beta chains of fibrinogen stimulate proliferation of human fibroblasts, Journal of Cell Science 104 409-413.

24.   R.M. Senior, W.F. Skogen, G.L. Griffin, G.D. Wilner. (1986) Effects of fibrinogen derivatives upon the inflammatory response. Studies with human fibrinopeptide B, Journal of Clinical Investigation 77 1014-1019.

25.   D. Manwaring, D. Thorning, P.W. Curreri. (1978)Mechanisms of acute pulmonary dysfunction induced by fibrinogen degradation product D, Surgery 84 45-54.

26.   D.T. Eitzman, R.D. McCoy, X. Zheng, W.P. Fay, T. Shen, D. Ginsburg, R.H. Simon. (1996) Bleomycin-induced pulmonary fibrosis in transgenic mice that either lack or overexpress the murine plasminogen activator inhibitor-1 gene, Journal of Clinical Investigation 97 232-237.

27.   M. Benezra, I. Vlodavsky, R. Ishai Michaeli, G. Neufeld, R. Bar Shavit. (1993) Thrombin-induced release of active basic fibroblast growth factor-heparan sulfate complexes from subendothelial extracellular matrix, Blood 81 3324-3331.

28.   R.J. Grand, A.S. Turnell, P.W. Grabham. (1996) Cellular consequences of thrombin-receptor activation, Biochemical Journal 313 353-368.

29.   O. Dery, C.U. Corvera, M. Steinhoff, N.W. Bunnett. (1998) Proteinase-activated receptors: novel mechanisms of signalling by serine proteases, American Journal of Physiology 274 C1429-C1452.

30.   T.K. Vu, D.T. Hung, V.I. Wheaton, S.R. Coughlin. (1991) Molecular cloning of a functional thrombin receptor reveals a novel proteolytic mechanism of receptor activation, Cell 64 1057-1068.

31.   H. Ishihara, A.J. Connolly, D. Zeng, M.L. Kahn, Y.W. Zheng, C. Timmons, T. Tram, S.R. (1997)Coughlin. Protease-activated receptor 3 is a second thrombin receptor in humans, Nature 386 502-506.

32.   W.F. Xu, H. Andersen, T.E. Whitmore, S.R. Presnell, D.P. Yee, A. Ching, T. Gilbert, E.W. Davie, D.C. Foster. (1998)Cloning and characterization of human protease-activated receptor 4, Proceedings of the National Academy of Sciences USA 95 6642-6646.

33.   D.T. Hung, T.K. Vu, V.I. Wheaton, K. Ishii, S.R. Coughlin. (1992) Cloned platelet thrombin receptor is necessary for thrombin-induced platelet activation, Journal of Clinical Investigation 89 1350-1353.

34.   A.J. Connolly, H. Ishihara, M.L. Kahn, R.V. Farese, Jr., S.R. Coughlin. (1996) Role of the thrombin receptor in development and evidence for a second receptor, Nature 381 516-519.

35.   M.L. Kahn, Y.W. Zheng, W. Huang, V. Bigornia, D. Zeng, S. Moff, R.V. Farese, Jr., C. Tam, S.R. Coughlin. (1998) A dual thrombin receptor system for platelet activation, Nature 394 690-694.

36.   H. Lum, T.T. Andersen, A. Siflinger Birnboim, C. Tiruppathi, M.S. Goligorsky, J.W. Fenton, 2d, A.B. Malik. (1993)Thrombin receptor peptide inhibits thrombin-induced increase in endothelial permeability by receptor desensitization, Journal of Cellular Biology 120 1491-1499.

37.   G. Cirino, C. Cicala, M.R. Bucci, L. Sorrentino, J.M. Maraganore, S.R. Stone. (1996) Thrombin functions as an inflammatory mediator through activation of its receptor, Journal of Experimental Medicine 183 821-827.

38.   S.K. Lo, M.B. Perlman, G.D. Niehaus, A.B. Malik. (1985)Thrombin-induced alterations in lung fluid balance in awake sheep, Journal of Applied Physiology 58 1421-1427.

39.   R. Bar-Shavit, A. Kahn, G.D. Wilner, J.W. Fenton, 2d. (1983) Monocyte chemotaxis: stimulation by specific exosite region in thrombin, Science 220 728-731.

40.   L.E. Sower, C.J. Froelich, D.H. Carney, J.W. Fenton, G.R. Klimpel. (1995) Thrombin induces IL-6 production in fibroblasts and epithelial cells. Evidence for the involvement of the seven-transmembrane domain (STD) receptor for alpha-thrombin, Journal of Immunology 155 895-901.

41.   A. Ueno, K. Murakami, K. Yamanouchi, M. Watanabe, T. Kondo. (1996) Thrombin stimulates production of interleukin-8 in human umbilical vein endothelial cells, Immunology 88 76-81.

42.   Y. Sugama, C. Tiruppathi, K. Offakidevi, T.T. Andersen, J.W. Fenton, 2d, A.B. Malik. (1992)Thrombin-induced expression of endothelial P-selectin and intercellular adhesion molecule-1: a mechanism for stabilizing neutrophil adhesion, *Journal of Cell Biology* **119** 935-944.

43.   K. Yokoi, N. Mukaida, A. Harada, Y. Watanabe, K. Matsushima. (1997 Prevention of endotoxaemia-induced acute respiratory distress syndrome-like lung injury in rabbits by a monoclonal antibody to IL-8, *Laboratory Investigation* **76** 375-384.

44.   L.B. Chen, J.M. Buchanan. (1975) Mitogenic activity of blood components. I. Thrombin and prothrombin, *Proceedings of the National Academy of Sciences USA* **72** 131-135.

45.   C.A. McNamara, I.J. Sarembock, L.W. Gimple, J.W. Fenton, 2d, S.R. Coughlin, G.K. Owens. (1993) Thrombin stimulates proliferation of cultured rat aortic smooth muscle cells by a proteolytically activated receptor, *Journal of Clinical Investigation* **91** 94-98.

46.   I.J. Sarembock, S.D. Gertz, L.W. Gimple, R.M. Owen, E.R. Powers, W.C. Roberts. (1991) Effectiveness of recombinant desulphatohirudin in reducing restenosis after balloon angioplasty of atherosclerotic femoral arteries in rabbits, *Circulation* **84** 232-243.

47.   N.A. Nelken, S.J. Soifer, J. O'Keefe, T.K. Vu, I.F. Charo, S.R. Coughlin. (1992) Thrombin receptor expression in normal and atherosclerotic human arteries, *Journal of Clinical Investigation* **90** 1614-1621.

48.   J. Trejo, A.J. Connolly, S.R. Coughlin. (1996) The cloned thrombin receptor is necessary and sufficient for activation of mitogen-activated protein kinase and mitogenesis in mouse lung fibroblasts. Loss of responses in fibroblasts from receptor knockout mice, *Journal of Biological Chemistry* **271** 21536-21541.

49.   T. Ohba, Y. Takase, M. Ohhara, R. Kasukawa. (1996) Thrombin in the synovial fluid of patients with rheumatoid arthritis mediates proliferation of synovial fibroblast-like cells by induction of platelet derived growth factor, *Journal of Rheumatology* **23** 1505-1511.

50.   E.M. Scarpati, P.E. DiCorleto. (1996) Identification of a thrombin response element in the human platelet-derived growth factor B-chain (c-sis) promoter, *Journal of Biological Chemistry* **271** 3025-3032.

51.   K.E. Dawes, A.J. Gray, G.J. Laurent. (1993) Thrombin stimulates fibroblast chemotaxis and replication, *European Journal of Cell Biology* **61** 126-130.

52.   Y.H. Kang, V.P. Kedar, R.K. Maheshwari. (1991) Thrombin stimulation of synthesis and secretion of fibronectin by human A549 epithelial cells and mouse LB fibroblasts, *Journal of Histochemistry and Cytochemistry* **39** 413-423.

53.   F. Peracchia, A. Tamburro, M. Zanni, D. Rotilio. (1994) Effects of thrombin and thrombin peptide activating receptor (SFLLRN) on proteoglycan synthesis and distribution in human endothelial cells, *Biochemical and Biophysical Research Communications* **205** 1625-1631.

54.   R.C. Chambers, K. Dabbagh, R.J. McAnulty, A.J. Gray, O.P. Blanc Brude, G.J. Laurent. (1998) Thrombin stimulates fibroblast procollagen production via proteolytic activation of protease-activated receptor 1, *Biochemical Journal* **333** 121-127.

55.   K. Dabbagh, G.J. Laurent, P.J. McAnulty, R.C. Chambers. (1998) Thrombin stimulates smooth muscle cell procollagen synthesis and mRNA levels via a PAR-1 mediated mechanism, *Thrombosis and Haemostasis* **79** 405-409.

56.   E. Papadimitriou, V.G. Manolopoulos, G.T. Hayman, M.E. Maragoudakis, B.R. Unsworth, J.W. Fenton, P.I. Lelkes. (1997) Thrombin modulates vectorial secretion of extracellular matrix proteins in cultured endothelial cells, *American Journal of Physiology* **272** C1112-C1122.

57.   B.K. Pilcher, D.W. Kim, D.H. Carney, J.J. Tomasek. (1994) Thrombin stimulates fibroblast-mediated collagen lattice contraction by its proteolytically activated receptor, *Experimental Cell Research* **211** 368-373.

58.   E. Duhamel-Clerin, C. Orvain, F. Lanza, J.P. Cazenave, C. Klein-Soyer. (1997) Thrombin receptor-mediated increase of two matrix metalloproteinases, MMP-1 and MMP-3, in human endothelial cells, *Arteriosclerosis, Thrombosis and Vascular Biology* **17** 1931-1938.

59.   D.H. Carney, R .Mann, W.R. Redin, S.D. Pernia, D. Berry, J.P. Heggers, P.G. Hayward, M.C. Robson, J. Christie, C. Annable, et al, (1992) Enhancement of incisional wound healing and neovascularization in normal rats by thrombin and synthetic thrombin receptor-activating peptides, *Journal of Clinical Investigation* **89** 1469-77.

60.   A.J. Connolly, D.Y. Suh, T.K. Hunt, S.R. Coughlin. (1997) Mice lacking the thrombin receptor, PAR-1, have normal skin wound healing, *American Journal of Pathology* **151** 1199-1204.

61.   I.J. Sarembock, S.D. Gertz, L.W. Gimple, R.M. Owen, E.R. Powers, W.C. Roberts. (1991) Effectiveness of recombinant desulphatohirudin in reducing restenosis after balloon angioplasty of atherosclerotic femoral arteries in rabbits, *Laboratory Investigation* **84** 232-243.

62.   M. Takada, H. Tanaka, T. Yamada, O. Ito, M. Kogushi, M. Yanagimachi, T. Kawamura, T. Musha, F. Yoshida, M. Ito, H. Kobayashi H, S. Yoshitake, I. Saito. (1998) Antibody to thrombin receptor inhibits neointimal smooth muscle cell accumulation without causing inhibition of platelet

aggregation or altering hemostatic parameters after angioplasty in rat. *Circulation Research* **82** 980-987.

63.   L.F. Brass. (1997) Thrombin receptor antagonists: a work in progress, Coronary Artery Disease **8** 49-58.

Neutrophil- and macrophage-derived proteases in chronic obstructive pulmonary disease and acute respiratory distress syndrome

Terry D. Tetley

Department of Respiratory Medicine, Charing Cross Hospital, Imperial College School of Medicine, London, UK

1   Introduction.

Pulmonary fibrosis and emphysema are peripheral lung diseases in which the connective tissue scaffold is totally, and irreversibly, reconstructed. To all intents and purposes, they appear to represent the opposite ends of a spectrum. Thus, in emphysema the gross appearance is of loss of tissue and formation of holes, whereas in fibrosis there is a massive increase in connective tissue which, in diffuse alveolar fibrosis, means a loss of airspaces due to invasion by fibrotic tissue. A major feature of emphysema is reduced elastic recoil which, particularly when associated with small airways disease, leads to obstruction of the airways. Although emphysema involves loss of connective tissue, microscopical examination reveals regions of fibrosis in the alveolar walls [1]; in addition, in chronic obstructive pulmonary disease (COPD) which can include small airways disease and bronchitis, part of the airways obstruction is due to diffuse fibrosis in the airway wall [1]. In diffuse alveolar fibrosis that occurs in the acute respiratory distress syndrome (ARDS), the increase in collagen deposition leads to stiffening of lung tissue and restrictive lung disease. While emphysema is most commonly associated with cigarette smoking or occupational dust exposure, ARDS can be triggered by a number of factors including septicaemia and endotoxin release by gram negative organisms, trauma and aspiration.

An early host response to inhaled toxins, organic and inorganic material is sequestration of circulating neutrophils and monocytes into the lung. An important component of the defence strategy of these inflammatory cells is generation proteolytic enzymes [2,3]. The activity of these enzymes is usually strictly controlled by containment and compartmentalisation, as well as inhibition via the pulmonary antiprotease screen, to achieve maximal defence, repair and resolution of the inflammation. However, when these controlling mechanisms fail, excessive protease activity can be cytotoxic, destroy the cellular and extracellular framework of the lung and potentiate inflammation, leading to a vicious, often uncontrollable, cycle of pathological events.

2   Pulmonary inflammation in chronic obstructive pulmonary disease (COPD).

Neutrophils are increased throughout the airway lumen of smokers, and especially so in those with COPD. They are rarely present within the interstitium or mucosa. The proportion of neutrophils in bronchoalveolar lavage (BAL; i.e. below the 4th or 5th airway generation) from COPD subjects increases from less than 5% to between 10 and 30% of the total [4]. Together with the 5-10-fold increase in total BAL cell number, this is a significant change. However, the majority of BAL neutrophils are collected during recovery of the first aliquot of lavage fluid, suggesting that these cells are primarily of airway, rather than alveolar, origin [4, 5, 6]. Investigation of the inflammatory cell profile of sputum and induced sputum (i.e. from conducting airways) from smokers and smokers with COPD shows very high proportions of neutrophils, from 30% in non-smokers, increasing to 70% in those with COPD [7,8,9]. The remainder of the cells are largely macrophages. As the total cell number in these secretions increases about 6-fold [9], the overall increase in number and predominance of neutrophils is likely to be clinically significant in conducting airways. In contrast, macrophages are the predominant cell in the lumen of the alveoli [10], respiratory bronchioles and small airways [11], the major sites of panacinar and centrilobular emphysema and small airways disease, respectively [1]. Furthermore, macrophages also predominate, while lymphocytes and mast cells are elevated, in the alveolar [1,12], bronchial and airway wall of smokers and subjects with COPD [1].

These findings implicate macrophages rather than neutrophils as the source of destructive enzymes in small airways disease and emphysema in smokers, whereas neutrophils may target the conducting airways and trigger bronchitis. However, recent *in vivo* studies illustrate the potent effect of cigarette smoke on bone marrow neutrophil release and sequestration of these cells to the pulmonary capillary bed [13]. Since these younger neutrophils are less deformable, and cigarette smoke inhibits neutrophil deformability, enhancing neutrophil trapping in the lung [14], it seems unlikely that neutrophils are entirely uninvolved in the pathological processes that occur in the distal lung. Neutrophils may contribute to alveolar and bronchial damage first in the capillaries prior to migration into the alveoli, but are then rapidly sequestered from the alveolar region into the airways, due to a gradient of chemotactic factors such as interleukin 8, which is elevated and highly concentrated in sputum [8] and bronchial lavage [6] from smokers and subjects with COPD. This hypothesis is strengthened by the finding that IL8 concentration correlates with neutrophil numbers in these secretions, a relationship that was not seen in peripheral lung secretions [6]. There is a striking correlation between increased airway neutrophil number, reduced lung function and COPD [7, 15], which is in stark contrast to the association between elevated macrophages in the alveolar wall of smokers with mild to moderate emphysema and in regions of small airways disease [10,11]. Thus, the pathology of emphysema and COPD is likely to reflect the action of a spectrum of proteolytic enzymes released by both macrophages and neutrophils, possibly at different sites and in different quantities to provide varying profiles of protease activity [2]. As the name suggests, COPD is a chronic disease that develops over years and affects individuals in middle to late life.

3   Pulmonary inflammation in acute lung injury and ARDS.

The hallmark of the early inflammation that occurs during acute lung injury and development of ARDS is a rapid, overwhelming influx of neutrophils, increasing from less than 5% of the total in BAL from normal subjects to 70% or more in BAL from patients with acute lung injury [16, 17]. Absolute numbers of macrophages are relatively normal, or less than normal, suggesting specific enrolment of neutrophils to the lung and possibly inhibition of macrophage recruitment. Unlike COPD, which consists of a number of pathologies at different levels of the respiratory tract, inflammation during acute lung injury is diffuse and affects the distal, alveolar-capillary wall of the lung. Acute lung injury involves an early edema, atelectasis, inflammation and, in ARDS, fibrosis. BAL neutrophil numbers correlate with total protein levels, clinical measures of lung injury and development of ARDS [16], suggesting a direct relationship between neutrophil activation and lung injury. Immediate release of neutrophil chemokines such as IL8 and other pro-inflammatory cytokines [18] are a feature of acute lung injury that progresses to ARDS. However, the fact that ARDS can occur in subjects with neutropenia suggests that neutrophils are not essential for development of ARDS.

The early injury leading to ARDS is believed to reflect damage to both the endothelial and epithelial cells. As in cigarette smoke induced injury, sequestration of neutrophils in acute lung injury may be the consequence of triggered release from the bone marrow, and entrapment of young neutrophils in the pulmonary capillary bed, and endothelial damage prior to transit into the airspaces [19]. This damage has been ascribed to proteolytic rather than oxidative events [20]. However, the critical difference, both quantitatively and over time, in the pattern of neutrophil recruitment during acute lung injury and cigarette smoking will, at least in part, contribute to the differences in the time course and pathology of the disease processes.

4   Inflammatory cell proteases.

The first clue that inflammatory cell proteases might be involved in connective tissue damage and lung diseases emerged when alpha 1-antitrypsin (alpha 1-proteinase inhibitor; PI) deficiency was associated with early onset emphysema [21]. PI is an inhibitor of neutrophil elastase, which, as the name implies, cleaves elastin and this, alongside the fact that the enzyme is stored in neutrophil granules at high concentrations (1-3pmol), lends credence to its import in emphysema. In addition, intratracheal neutrophil elastase will induce a condition similar to emphysema in experimental animals. Consequently, the possible central role of neutrophil elastase in the pathology of emphysema has attracted the attention of researchers for more than thirty years [22, 23]. However, most smokers have normal PI levels and there is accumulating evidence to suggest that the pathology seen in emphysema is more likely to be due to a combination of proteolytic enzymes which act in synergy, to great effect [2,3].

In recent years, a wide range of inflammatory cell-derived proteases with the potential to degrade extracellular matrix have been investigated in a number of lung diseases, including COPD and pulmonary fibrosis, on the premise that modified protease action contributes to the connective tissue abnormalities that occur in these diseases. Proteases that target the interstitial collagens and elastin, which are particularly resistant proteins, have received much attention. Complementary, often parallel, studies have examined the possible contribution of modified antiprotease protection to these events.

5   Neutrophil proteases.

In addition to neutrophil elastase, neutrophils store two other serine proteases cathepsin G and proteinase 3 in the primary, azurophil, granules [2,3]. They are approximately 25-30kDa. Neutrophils also store at least two matrix metalloproteinases, neutrophil collagenase (75kDa; secondary granules) and gelatinase B (92kDa; tertiary granules) [2,3]. All these enzymes may be released during neutrophil activation, react efficiently at neutral pH and can degrade all the major constituents of the extracellular matrix - elastin, interstitial and basement membrane collagens, laminin, fibronectin and proteoglycans. It seems unlikely that release of these enzymes by neutrophils during inflammation is entirely exclusive, particularly if the cells undergo necrosis rather than apoptosis.

6   Matrix metalloproteinases.

Both neutrophils and macrophages release metalloproteinases - enzymes that require a metal ion - Zn^{2+} and Ca^{2+} - at the catalytic site for activity [3]. Unlike neutrophils, macrophages synthesise and secrete metalloproteinases as required and when activated. These enzymes are released in a latent, inactive form. Originally named for their functional properties, the family is large and the nomenclature has now been simplified to matrix metalloproteinase (MMP) followed by a number usually denoting the chronology of its discovery. The interstitial collagens, types I, II and III are the most resistant to proteolysis and are targeted by interstitial collagenase, MMP1 (55kDa; released from stromal cells and macrophages) and neutrophil collagenase, MMP8 (75kDa). Recently, gelatinase A, MMP2 (72kDa), has been shown to degrade type I collagen, as has a membrane bound, membrane type matrix metalloproteinase, MT1-MMP [24]. The gelatinases, MMP2 (released mostly from stromal cells) and MMP 9 (92kDa; gelatinase B; released by neutrophils and macrophages) degrade denatured interstitial collagens, gelatin, basement membrane collagens, elastin and proteoglycans. Macrophage metalloelastase, MMP12 (55kDa), degrades elastin and fibronectin.

Structurally, MMPs are highly homologous [3, 25]. Most consist of three domains. An N-terminal propeptide domain which folds to mask the active site of a second, catalytic domain containing the Zn^{2+} binding site. The C-terminal domain confers substrate specificity and, in gelatinases, enables binding to substrate and hence specificity of reactivity. The C-terminal is also the binding region for the tissue inhibitors of metalloproteinases, TIMP1 and TIMP2. Latent MMPs contain a conserved cysteine residue within the N-terminal domain that interacts with the Zn^{2+} binding site of the catalytic domain, preventing reactivity. Chelation by organomercurials, oxidation or proteolysis, of the cysteine residue frees the reactive site, leading to autolytic cleavage of the propeptide and generation of active enzyme. The enzyme may continue to undergo autolytic or proteolytic cleavage to a smaller, inactive molecule.

7   Macrophage lysosomal cysteine proteases.

Macrophages also store proteases in lysosomes [26]. Although lysosomal cysteine proteases are most effective at acid pH, to dissolve internalised organic particles and micro-organisms, some cysteine proteases operate at neutral pH and extracellularly. Macrophages can channel these enzymes to the cell surface within endosomal/lysosomal structures to enable pericellular proteolysis that is protected from inhibitors. The cysteine proteases, cathepsins K, S and L, are all capable of degrading insoluble elastin. Although, compared to neutrophil elastase and all other elastases, cathepsin K is the most potent elastase at acid pH [see 26], it is unstable at neutral pH. In contrast, cathepsin S, which is also a potent elastinolytic enzyme at acid pH, is less active, but remains stable, at neutral pH. Nevertheless, even at neutral pH it has similar reactivity to neutrophil elastase and gelatinase A (MMP2), and greater activity than proteinase 3, macrophage metalloelastase and gelatinase B (MMP9). *In vitro* studies support the suggestion that mobilisation of cathepsins L, S and K [26,27] results in extracellular elastin degradation. Importantly, in addition to elastin, cathepsins K, S and L degrade collagen and gelatin. Macrophage cathepsins are therefore likely to contribute to connective tissue remodelling during inflammation and may be significant in pulmonary connective tissue pathology.

8   Synergistic action of inflammatory cell proteases.

Parallel release of proteases by neutrophils and macrophages at the same site has a number of implications. Neutrophil elastase has broad substrate specificity; e.g. it stimulates chemokine release from pulmonary epithelial cells so potentiating inflammation, it activates complement which triggers neutrophil activation and migration, and it can degrade surfactant apoproteins so compromising immunological and surface tension reducing functions of surfactant. Significantly, neutrophil elastase (and possibly other serine proteases) can activate at least one of the gelatinases, gelatinase B (MMP9) [28], and possibly other metalloproteinases, as well as inactivate TIMPs [29], thus enhancing proteolytic potential. In addition, chlorinated oxidants (e.g. HOCl) generated during activation of neutrophils activate gelatinase B (MMP9) and interstitial neutrophil collagenase (MMP8) by oxidative mechanisms [30]. Gelatinase B (MMP9) can, in turn, potentiate the activity of neutrophil collagenase (MMP8). The release and activation of neutrophil and macrophage proteases is normally strictly regulated by controlled, compartmentalised release, and specific inhibition. Overwhelming inflammation with inadequate inhibition is likely to result in a complex cocktail of extracellular proteolytic enzymes. Thus, this situation is likely to lend itself to amplification of protease activity due to activation of latent metalloproteinases and inactivation of their inhibitors by serine proteases. In addition, metalloproteinases cleave and inactivate the major serum serine protease inhibitor, PI [2]. Together with release of oxidative molecules by inflammatory cells, which may also activate metalloproteinases and inactivate PI, the protease-antiprotease balance becomes unstable, ultimately favouring proteases.

9   Pulmonary antiprotease screen.

9.1   Inhibitors of serine proteases.

In the lung, this antiprotease screen mainly consists of serum-derived PI, a member of the serpin (SERine Protease INhibitor) family, and locally produced inhibitors. PI is synthesised in small quantities by epithelial cells and macrophages, but it is difficult to assess the relevance of this when compared to the amount of PI that transudes from the blood, which accounts for virtually all of that present in lung tissue. PI inhibits neutrophil elastase, cathepsin G and proteinase 3 [31, 32]. Epithelial cells synthesise and secrete secretory leukoprotease inhibitor, SLPI (also called bronchial mucus protease inhibitor, antileukoprotease and mucus protease inhibitor) as well as elafin. Both these inhibitors are of low molecular weight compared to PI, which is 52kDa. SLPI is 12kDa, while elafin is 6kDa. SLPI inhibits neutrophil elastase and cathepsin G but not proteinase 3 [see 33]. The low molecular weight of SLPI and elafin enables access to pericellular sites that PI cannot target. In addition, SLPI is released both apically and basally from epithelial cells, and will therefore target interstitial and luminal serine proteases. Little is known about the amount of elafin in lung secretions, although one group have suggested that it exists at relatively high levels [34], while another could detect no elafin activity in bronchoalveolar lavage

[35]. In contrast, SLPI has been detected in secretions throughout the respiratory tract. In comparison to PI, it contributes over 95% of the inhibitory profile in nasal secretions, 80-90% of that in the large airways, gradually contributing less in the smaller airways and peripheral lung, where it is detected at 10-20% compared to PI [33]. There are some important differences in the activity of PI and SLPI, which appear to act in concert [33]. For example, PI is an irreversible inhibitor of neutrophil elastase and does not inhibit the enzyme when it is bound to insoluble substrate such as elastin. In contrast, SLPI is a reversible inhibitor of neutrophil elastase and will inhibit neutrophil elastase even when bound to elastin. PI will, however, displace neutrophil elastase from SLPI, irreversibly bind to neutrophil elastase and clear it from its site of action i.e. the lung. Displacement of SLPI-bound neutrophil elastase and clearance by PI leaves SLPI to continue to mop up substrate-bound neutrophil elastase. Less is known about the role of elafin in clearing serine proteases from the lung.

9.2   Alpha1-antichymotrypsin.

The major inhibitor of cathepsin G is alpha1-antichymotrypsin, which like PI, is a serpin and transudes into the lung from serum, although small amounts may be synthesised by resident lung cells [36]. It is normally present at low levels, reflecting its serum concentration. However, as an acute phase protein, its level can rise five-fold in response to injury and infection, and a polymorphism has been associated with COPD, implicating cathepsin G in the pathology of this condition.

9.3   Matrix metalloproteinase inhibitors.

The activity of MMPs is closely regulated by tissue inhibitors of metalloproteinases (TIMP) which are normally synthesised and secreted alongside the metalloproteinases. Although 4 TIMPs have been described, most is known about the activity of TIMP1 (29kDa), TIMP2 (21kDa) and TIMP3 (21kDa); TIMP1 is glycosylated, the unglycosylated form having the same molecular weight as TIMPs 1 and 2 [3,36]. TIMP can react with the active site of the activated MMP. TIMP also binds tightly to the N-terminal of the latent MMP so that it cannot access its substrate. As mentioned earlier, the gelatinases, MMP2 and MMP9, are secreted as a complex with TIMP [3,25,36], providing protection from proteolytic degradation by other proteases and extending the half life of the enzyme. The exact processes by which these complexes work is currently under intensive investigation. Clearly, latent MMP bound to TIMP will not only have to be activated, it, or the active site, will also have to be free of its inhibitor before proteolysis can take place. Interestingly, TIMP2 release appears to be more constitutive in nature, while TIMP 1 and 3 can be regulated by various stimuli [36]. Since TIMPs are commonly synthesised in parallel with their MMPs, increased MMP activity will partly depend on specific up-regulation of MMP synthesis, and/or down-regulation of TIMP synthesis; reduced MMP activity is likely to be the converse of this.

9.4   Cysteine proteinase inhibitors.

Family 2 cystatins are the most abundant secreted, extracellular inhibitors of cysteine proteases. Family 1 cystatins operate intra- and extracellularly, while family 3 cystatins, kininogens, are the most abundant serum inhibitors [36]. Family 2 cystatins are likely to be the most significant in terms of controlling extracellular cysteine proteases [26, 36] and are enriched in epithelial secretions. Like SLPI, they are small molecules of about 12kDa. The mode of inhibition of cysteine proteases is more complex than that of serine protease inhibitors, via multiple sites. Nevertheless, inhibition is irreversible. Recently, a protease inhibitor, (squamous cell carcinoma antigen; SSCA), belonging to the serpin family, has been described which is also a potent inhibitor of cathepsin K, S and L. SSCA has been localised to the ciliated cells of the conducting airways, mostly intracellular [see 26]. Its role is unclear, but it may be important in protecting the airways from unrestricted cysteine protease activity.

9.5   Alpha 2-macroglobulin.

Alpha 2-macroglobulin is a large tetramer of four identical 180kDa molecules [36]. It inhibits most proteinases by steric hindrance, containing a bait region on each subunit. Cleavage of the bait region results in a conformational change and entrapment of the protease within the tetramer. The change in inhibitor conformation during this process also exposes a cell receptor binding site, binding of which leads to internalisation and lysosomal degradation of the inhibitor and caged protease. Alpha 2-macroglobulin is present in serum at high concentrations and due to its high molecular weight only transudes into lung tissue in any quantity when there is endothelial and epithelial damage. However, many cells synthesise this inhibitor, although it isn't clear how relevant these sources are to the pulmonary inhibitor screen.

10   Inflammatory cell proteases.

10.1   In emphysema.

Although both levels and activity of human BAL neutrophil elastase have been positively associated with emphysema [2,37] it has proven difficult to illustrate its presence in the interstitium, although elastin degradation products are elevated in the plasma and urine of COPD subjects [23]. This may reflect the chronic nature of the condition with a constant, small but clinically significant increase in elastolysis. On the other hand, in man neutrophil elastase may contribute only a minor part of the elastinolytic process known to occur in this disease, being primarily involved in the generation of pro-inflammatory mediators and potentiation of the disease. Other relevant proteases include collagenase; over expression of human collagenase in mice gives rise to an emphysema-like condition where the major connective tissue defect was loss of interstitial collagen with normal elastin [38]. However, it is possible in this model that the problem reflects a developmental problem due to insufficient structural matrix to enable normal alveolarisation. In support of increased collagenase and collagen degradation as a factor in emphysema, guinea pigs exposed to 20 cigarettes a day for up to 8 weeks developed emphysematous changes which were associated with loss of lung collagen [39] and increased collagenase activity. Collagenase mRNA expression was increased, especially in alveolar macrophages, which also immunostained strongly for collagenase, suggesting that these cells played a primary role in the development of emphysema. Unfortunately, elastinolytic activity was not assessed and it is unclear whether part of the pathology reflected metalloproteinase inhibition of PI and increased serine elastase activity.

Macrophage metalloelastase (MMP12) may contribute to emphysema [40]. Although this enzyme won't degrade interstitial collagen, it degrades elastin and most other matrix components. Mice genetically deficient in macrophage metalloelastase did not, whereas macrophage elastase sufficient mice did, develop emphysema when exposed to cigarette smoke for up to six months [40]. There was no macrophage infiltration of lung tissue in macrophage elastase-deficient mice, suggesting that this enzyme is important during cell migration. Even when these deficient mice received intratracheal monocyte chemoattractant protein1 to encourage macrophage recruitment, there was no emphysema, implicating the macrophage metalloelastase as the sole enzyme responsible for emphysema in this model. However, the significance of the human equivalent, human macrophage metalloelastase, HME (MMP12), in human emphysema has not been confirmed - BAL macrophages from normal or emphysematous subjects do not appear to express mRNA for macrophage metalloelastase[41].

In contrast, investigation of macrophage MMP mRNA expression and protein production revealed upregulation of interstitial collagenase (MMP1) and gelatinase B (MMP9) by human macrophages from emphysematous patients [41]. In addition, these cells released neutrophil-derived serine proteases *in vitro*, supporting macrophage release of internalised neutrophil elastase as a contributory mechanism in the pathology in emphysema. Parallel studies on the acellular bronchoalveolar lavage from these subjects confirmed the presence of elevated neutrophil elastase, especially in the smokers' BAL [37]; in addition, collagenolytic activity and the proenzyme form of neutrophil-derived gelatinase (MMP9) increased.

Examination of human emphysematous lung tissue homogenate showed no differences in immunological levels of neutrophil elastase, but highlighted increased levels of both gelatinase A (MMP2) and gelatinase B (MMP9) as well as activity against elastin, gelatin and collagen, in association with emphysema [42]. Gelatinase A (MMP2) was present both as latent and activated enzyme. The latter was believed to be due to increased membrane-type matrix metalloproteinase, MT1-MMP, which activates gelatinase A (MMP2) and can also degrade type I, II and III collagen. The gelatinase A (MMP2)/MT1-MMP activation mechanism requires TIMP2, which was also found to be elevated. Co-ordinated activation of gelatinase A (MMP2) by the membrane-type of MMP and independent action of MMP2 and MT1-MMP could therefore account for a significant proportion of the matrix degradation observed in emphysema. These studies in humans implicate both serine and metalloproteases in the later stages (repair?) of emphysema; however, it is difficult to study early disease processes, as emphysema is largely undiagnosed until the disease becomes clinically significant.

Neutrophil elastase can only be localised to elastin in emphysematous tissue when albumin is used as a blocking agent [43]. When an appropriate blocking agent, non-immune serum from the same species as the second antibody, is used, neutrophil elastase is present in neutrophil granules but not on elastic tissue [44]. Unlike the metalloproteinases, which may bind to extracellular matrix components, there is little evidence that this is true for neutrophil elastase. In support of this, subsequent studies imply that neutrophil elastase degrades the edges of the elastic tissue [45], and it is suggested that the enzyme is swiftly displaced and cleared from the active site by SLPI and PI [33]. SLPI binds to interstitial elastin and may prevent long-term binding of neutrophil elastase. Inadequate SLPI may enable elevated elastolysis during neutrophil inflammation and development of emphysema. For example, when ten apparently healthy smokers' BALs were analysed for SLPI levels and activity, one subject without SLPI, and one with inactive SLPI, were found to have subclinical emphysema, detected by computerised tomography [47]. None of the remainder had emphysema or were deficient in SLPI.

There are no extensive investigations of macrophage lysosomal cathepsins in emphysema. A recent study of BAL from smokers with subclinical emphysema (i.e. airspace enlargement without functional change) indicated that the immunological level of cathepsin L, but not activity, was elevated in these subjects [47]. Increased cathepsin L was accompanied by increased cystatin C inhibitor which may account for the lack of change in protease activity. Basal cathepsin K synthesis by macrophages is almost nil but both protein and mRNA increase approximately two-fold in macrophages from smokers [see 26]. These observations, the known potency of cathepsins K, L and S to degrade elastin and interstitial collagens, as well as the capacity of the macrophage to regulate and target cathepsin action, suggest that cathepsins are serious contenders for a pathological role in emphysema.

10.2   In COPD.

The possible contribution of proteases to the pathology of bronchioles, small and large airways in COPD has not been investigated in depth until recently. Many of these studies have been concerned with analysis of bronchial secretions, rather than tissue. Sputum and induced sputum provide samples from the large conducting airways but it is more difficult to sample small airways. However, presence of measurable elastolytic activity in sputum was found to be directly related to exacerbation of COPD [48]. Cathepsin G activity was also elevated. It is of interest that elevated elastase activity was unrelated to immunologic PI level, which was present in molar excess and should have inhibited free elastase. However, the inhibitory capacity of PI was not determined. The immunological level of SLPI on the other hand, was inversely related to elastase activity and therefore consistently low during exacerbation of COPD, suggesting that inhibition of elastase by SLPI is a significant controlling mechanism in the airways and that unrestricted elastase, contributes to COPD.

Analysis of sputum from subjects with COPD showed a direct correlation between elevated levels of gelatinase B (MMP9), neutrophil and macrophage numbers [49]. However, the enzyme was inactive, being present in only in its latent form. This may reflect increased TIMP1 which increased relatively more than gelatinase B (MMP9). The gelatinase B (MMP9)/TIMP1 ratio correlated inversely with FEV1, suggesting that gelatinase B (MMP9)/TIMP1 imbalance in favour of inhibitor may prevent extracellular matrix degradation by migratory cells, or triggering of growth factor release, and therefore contribute to airway wall fibrosis and obstruction in COPD.

10.3   In acute lung injury and ARDS.

Both BAL neutrophil elastase levels and collagenase activity have been positively associated with ARDS [50,51,52], as has serum neutrophil elastase levels [53]. The acute, massive influx of neutrophils in acute lung injury is accompanied by edema and increased plasma proteins, including PI and alpha 2-macroglobulin, into the alveoli, as well as increased local SLPI release. Consequently, although immunological levels of neutrophil elastase increase, it is only during severe cases, where the antiprotease screen is severely compromised, that free elastolytic activity can be detected. This may partly be due to oxidative inactivation of PI [54]. Nevertheless, neutrophil elastase may mediate the disease following pericellular release in close proximity to endothelial and epithelial cells, as well as basement membrane and extracellular matrix, during sequestration into the airspaces. Breaching of the alveolar-capillary basement membrane may precipitate increased permeability, invasion by interstitial cells followed by collagen deposition in the alveolar space and fibrosis. Apart from degradation of extracellular matrix, it seems likely that neutrophil elastase potentiates inflammation via activation of complement and generation of chemotactic agents.

There are few investigations of matrix metalloproteinases in humans with ARDS. Immunologic gelatinase B (MMP9) was found to be elevated in BAL from subjects with ARDS [17]. It was elevated in the early stages in both subjects at risk as well as those who progressed to ARDS. However, during the course of ARDS, gelatinase B (MMP9) levels remained elevated, but declined in those at risk whose condition had improved. Parallel analysis of TIMP1 showed a different pattern of change. Early in the disease process,

TIMP1 was most dramatically increased in those who developed ARDS, but fell steadily during the following 10 weeks. Thus, during the development of ARDS, the ratio of gelatinase B (MMP9) to TIMP1 increased in favour of gelatinase B (MMP9), suggesting that gelatinase B (MMP9) is involved in repair and remodelling rather than early damage. Interestingly, gelatinase B (MMP9) levels correlated with neutrophil levels rather than macrophages, illustrating the significance of neutrophil-derived products in the disease process.

In contrast, Delclaux and colleagues carried out a study of BAL proteinases during established ARDS, almost entirely related to the activity, rather than immunological level, of the enzymes [55]. They investigated the presence and activity of both gelatinases, A and B (MMP2, MMP9). The study was different to that of Ricou et al; one BAL was collected from subjects with ARDS with multiple organ failure (MOF), ARDS without MOF, MOF without ARDS, neither ARDS nor MOF. A striking finding was that activated BAL gelatinase A (MMP2) was discovered in 16 of 18 patients with ARDS, whether or not they had MOF, but not in any of the other patients. Approximately half the patients' BAL contained active as well as latent gelatinase B (MMP9); unlike gelatinase A (MMP2), this did not correlate with ARDS. Although both gelatinases increased per unit ARDS BAL (but not necessarily per unit of lung secretion, which was 4 times greater in ARDS BAL) the presence of activated gelatinase A (MMP2) suggests fibroblast and epithelial cell involvement during the fibrotic, repair stage. In contrast to Ricou et al, Delclaux et al suggest that inflammatory cell gelatinase B (MMP9) contributes to the early pathology and basement membrane degradation. There are clear differences between these studies, including time course, subject groups, gelatinase and TIMP assessment, which may account for the differences. Nevertheless, both studies highlight a role for gelatinases in the pathology of ARDS. It is suggested that in neutropenic patients with ARDS, gelatinases, with their broad substrate specificity, may be the primary proteolytic mediators.

It seems possible that neutrophil elastase and gelatinase B both contribute to development of ARDS, possibly at different stages of the disease, or by co-ordinated action. Although this mechanism of action has not been shown in humans with ARDS, gelatinase B increases in rodent models of endotoxin-induced lung injury. Use of specific neutrophil elastase inhibitors in one of these models illustrated the role of neutrophil elastase in the activation of gelatinase B, which could also be demonstrated *in vitro* [28]. Thus both classes of enzyme seem likely to contribute to acute lung injury prior to ARDS.

In rodent models of bleomycin-induced lung injury and fibrosis, which do not exactly mimic acute lung injury and ARDS in man, BAL gelatinase A (MMP2) increased early in the injury and predominated, although gelatinase B increased, though less so [56]. Release of gelatinase B may reflect the direct effect of bleomycin on macrophages [57]. A recent, comprehensive investigation of MMP and TIMP mRNA expression during bleomycin-induced lung damage in mice suggested specific up-regulation of MMPs since both gelatinase A (MMP2) and macrophage metalloelastase mRNA were elevated [58]. Gelatinase B (MMP9), and interstitial collagenase mRNA did not change. Bleomycin has also been demonstrated to stimulate rat lung tissue homogenate and alveolar macrophage cathepsins L, H, S and B [59]. Macrophages contained approximately five times as much cathepsin L activity as cathepsins H, S and B, which increased further, up to 4-fold after bleomycin, although it isn't clear whether this was assayed at acid or neutral pH. Cathepsin S was assayed at near neutral pH (6.5) and increased over 5-fold in macrophages following bleomycin. These animal studies support the predominant role of gelatinase A (MMP2) in the fibrotic response to lung injury; in addition they suggest macrophage-derived cathepsins could contribute to tissue damage and extracellular matrix remodelling during fibrosis. Since BAL alpha 2-macroglobulin and elastase inhibitory activity increased sharply following intratracheal bleomycin [59], and lung tissue TIMP1 (but not TIMP2 or TIMP3) mRNA expression increased [58], the successful action of inflammatory cell proteases will critically depend on regulated, site-directed release.

Unfortunately there are no immunolocalisation or mRNA hybridisation studies of MMPs and TIMPs in ARDS; however, gelatinase A and B (MMP2, MMP9), TIMP1 and TIMP2 have been immunolocalised in normal lung tissue and tissue from subjects with diffuse alveolar damage (DAD) and idiopathic pulmonary fibrosis (IPF) [60]. Both MMPs and both TIMPs were detected in epithelial cells, endothelial cells, macrophages and smooth muscle cells of normal lung. Fibroblasts contained only gelatinase A (MMP2). Both MMPs increased in epithelial cells and myofibroblasts of alveolar buds in IPF and DAD. Gelatinase B (MMP9) also increased in type II cells, fibroblasts (DAD and IPF) and macrophages I(IPF). Cellular TIMP1 and TIMP2 tended to increase in parallel to the MMPs. TIMP1 and TIMP2 were also located on the interstitial matrix and did not appear to change. Thus, both gelatinases and their inhibitors are up-regulated during remodelling of fibrotic tissues. A major drawback with this type of study is that it describes only one moment in the later stages of the disease and cannot elucidate early events. However, it is interesting to note that these MMPs and TIMPs are relatively ubiquitous in normal lung tissue.

11   Summary.

It seems unlikely that inflammatory cell-derived proteases do not contribute to development of COPD and ARDS. At present it is difficult to judge the relative importance of the different cell types and classes of enzymes to each disease. This very much reflects the early focus on neutrophil elastase and the difficulties associated with studies on metalloproteinases, including their latency and more complex mechanisms of action. Similarly, the evidence that cysteine proteinases contribute to these diseases reflects the diversity of action of this class of enzyme and possibly reluctance to acknowledge their matrix-degrading potential at neutral pH.

Accumulating evidence supports the possibility that different classes of enzyme operate in unison to potentiate proteolytic activity during inflammation. Virtually all of the enzymes studied increase at some stage, or in one lung compartment, in both COPD and ARDS. Neutrophil proteases, such as neutrophil elastase and gelatinase B (MMP9; also macrophage-derived) are commonly associated with early and acute events. However, chronic release and amplification of inflammation and metalloproteinase activity by these enzymes cannot be ignored. Interestingly, gelatinase A (MMP2) is elevated in both conditions but is likely to be derived mostly from non-inflammatory cells and reflect repair and remodelling. Regulation of gelatinase A (MMP2) activity by membrane-type proteases, which increase in parallel, is likely to be a significant controlling mechanism in terms of localising the site of enzyme activity. One suspects that it will prove difficult to establish the exact profile, pattern of release and contribution of individual inflammatory and resident cell proteases that occurs during COPD and ARDS. Most seem to be involved at some stage. COPD is problematic to study in the early stages when there are few symptoms; in addition, it progresses slowly over decades so that pathological changes cannot easily be detected. In contrast, ARDS progresses so rapidly that it also proves difficult to monitor.

In the absence of a clearly defined sequence of proteolytic events, one obvious approach to therapy would be to use a combination of inhibitors, which is beginning to prove successful in animal models of acute lung injury. Obviously, route of delivery and access to site of enzyme action will be crucial. In acute lung injury, it is possible that both intratracheal and intravenous delivery would be feasible. COPD on the other hand would require long-term treatment; inhalation therapy would be more feasible but might be complicated due to inefficient drug delivery. Thus, inhibitors must be able to target the site of action of the enzymes (e.g. be small enough, reach the peripheral lung). This type of therapeutic approach will require development of suitable antiproteolytic drug combinations and delivery systems.

References.

1.   Jeffrey PK. (1998) Structural and inflammatory changes in COPD: a comparison with asthma. *Thorax;* **53:**129-136
2.   Tetley TD. (1993) Proteinase imbalance: its role in lung disease. *Thorax;* **48:**560-565
3.   O'Connor CM, FitzGerald MX. (1994) Matrix metalloproteases and lung disease. *Thorax;* **49:**602-609
4.   Martin TR, Raghu G, Maunder RJ, Springmayer SC. (1985) The effects of chronic bronchitis and chronic air-flow obstruction on lung cell populations recovered by bronchoalveolar lavage. *Am Rev Respir Dis;* **132:**254-260
5.   Smith SF, Guz A, Winning AJ, Cooke NT, Burton GH, Tetley TD. (1988) Comparison of human lung surface protein profiles from the central and peripheral airways sampled using two regional lavage techniques *Eur Respir J;* **1:**792-800
6.   Mio T, Romberger DJ, Thompson AB, Robbins RA, Heires A, Rennard SI. (1997) Cigarette smoke induces interleukin-8 from bronchial epithelial cells. *Am. J. Respir. Crit. Care Med.;* **155:**1770-1776
7.   Stanescu D, Sanna A, Veriter C, Kostianev S, Calcagni PG, Fabbri LM, Maestrelli P. (1996) Airways obstruction, chronic expectoration, and rapid decline of FEV1 in smokers are associated with increased levels of sputum neutrophils. *Thorax;* **51:**267-271
8.   YamamotoC, Yoneda T, Yoshikawa M, Fu A, Tokuyama T, Tsukaguchi K, Narita N. (1997) Airway inflammation in COPD assessed by sputum levels of interleukin-8. *Chest;* **112:**505-510
9.   Keatings VM, Barnes PJ. (1997) Granulocyte activation markers in induced sputum: comparison between chronic obstructive pulmonary disease, asthma, and normal subjects. *Am J Crit Care Med;* **155:**449-453
10.   Hunninghake GW, Gadek JE, Kawanami O, Ferrans VJ, Crystal RG. (1979) Inflammatory and immune processes in the human lung in health and disease: evaluation by bronchoalveolar lavage. *Am J Pathol;* **97:**149-206
11.   Niewoehner DE, Kleinerman J, Rice DB. (1974) Pathologic changes in the peripheral airways of young cigarette smokers. *N. Engl. J. Med. ;* **291:**755-758
12.   Finkelstein R, Fraser RS, Cosio MG. (1995) Alveolar inflammation and its relationship to emphysema in smokers. *Am. J. Respir. Crit. Care Med.;* **152:**1666-1672
13.   Terashima T, Klut ME, English D, Hards J, Hogg JC, van Eeden SF. (1999) Cigarette smoking causes sequestration of polymorphonuclear leukocytes released from the bone marrow in lung microvessels. *Am J Respir Cell Moll Biol;* **20:**171-177.
14.   MacNee W, Wiggs B, Belzberg AS, Hogg JC. (1989) The effect of cigarette smoking on neutrophil kinetics in human lungs. *N. Engl. J. Med. ;* **321:**924-928
15.   Ronchi MC, Piragino C, Rosi E, Amendola M, Duranti R, Scano G. (1996) Role of sputum differential cell count in detecting airway inflammation in patients with chronic bronchial asthma or COPD. *Thorax;* **51:**1000-1004
16.   Weiland JE, Davis WB, Holter JF, Mohammed JR, Dorinsky PM, Gadek JE. (1986) Lung neutrophils in the adult respiratory distress syndrome, *Am Rev Respir Dis;* **133:**218-225
17.   Ricou B, Nicod L, Lacraz S, Welgus HG, Suter PM, Dayer J-M. (1996) Matrix metalloproteinase and TIMP in acute respiratory distress syndrome. *Am. J. Respir. Crit. Care Med.;* **154:**346-352
18.   Meduri GU, Kohler G, Headley S, Tolley E, Stentz F, Postlethwaite A. (1995) Inflammatory cytokines in the BAL of patients with ARDS. Persistent elevation over time predicts poor outcome. *Chest;* **108:**1303-1314
19.   Klut ME, Van Eeden SF, Whalen BA, Verburgt LM, English D, Hogg JC. (1996) Neutrophil activation and lung injury associated with chronic endotoxaemia in rabbits. *Exp. Lung Res.;* **22:**449-465
20.   Donovan KL, Davies M, Coles GA, Williams JD. (1994) Relative roles of elastase and reactive oxygen species in the degradation of human glomerular basement membrane by intact human neutrophils. *Kidney Int.;* **45:**1555-1561
21.   Laurell C-B, Eriksson S. (1963) The electrophoretic alpha 1-globulin pattern of serum in alpha 1-antitrypsin deficiency. *Scan J Clin Lab Invest;* **15:**132-40

22. Snider GL. (1992) Emphysema: The first two centuries. Part I. *Am Rev Respir Dis;* **146:**1334-44

23. Snider GL. (1992) Emphysema: The first two centuries. Part II. *Am Rev Respir Dis;* **146:**1615-22

24. Strongin AY, Collier I, Bannikov G, Marmer BL, Grant GA, Goldberg GI. (1995) Mechanism of cell surface activation of 72-kDa type IV collagenase. *J. Biol. Chem.;* **270:**5331-5338

25. Shapiro S. (1994) Elastolytic metalloproteinases produced by human mononuclear phagocytes. *Am. J. Respir. Crit. Care Med.;* **150:**S160-S164

26. Chapman HA, Riese RJ, Shi G-P. (1997) Emerging roles for cysteine proteases in human biology. *Annu Rev Physiol;* **59:**63-68

27. Reddy VY, Zhang Q-Y, Weiss SJ. (1995) Pericellular mobilization of the tissue-destructive cysteine proteases, cathepsins B, L, and S by human macrophages. *Proc. Natl. Acad. Sci. USA;* **92:**3849-3853

28. Ferry G, Lonchampt M, Pennel L, de Nanteuil G, Canet E, Tucker GC. (1997) Activation of MMP9 by neutrophil elastase in an in vivo model of acute lung injury. *FEBS Letts;* **402:**111-115

29. Okada Y, Watanabe S, Nakanishi I, Kishi J-I, Hayakawa T, Watorek W, Travis J, Nagase H. (1988) Inactivation of tissue inhibitor of metalloproteinases by neutrophil elastase and other serine proteinases. *FEBS Letts;* **229:**157-160

30. Peppin GJ, Weiss SJ. (1986) Activation of the endogenous metalloproteinase, gelatinase, by triggered human neutrophils. *Proc. Natl. Acad. Sci. USA;* **83:**4322-4326

31. Travis J. (1989) Alpha1-proteinase inhibitor deficiency. *In:* Lung cell biology. ed. Massaro M. New York: Marcell Decker; 1227-1246

32. Rao NV, Wehner NG, Marshall BC, Sturrock AB, Hueckstead TP, Rao GV, Gray BH, Hoidal JR. (1991) Proteinase -3 (PR3): A polymorphonuclear leukocyte serine proteinase. *Annals. N.Y. Acad. Sci.;* **624:**60-68

33. Bingle L & Tetley TD. (1996) Secretory leukoprotease inhibitor - partnering alpha-1 proteinase inhibitor to combat pulmonary inflammation. *Thorax;* **51:**1273-74

34. Tremblay GM, Sallenave JM, Israelassayag E, Cormier Y, Gauldie J. (1996) Elafin/elastase-specific inhibitor in bronchoalveolar lavage of normal subjects and farmers lung. *Am. J. Respir. Crit. Care Med.;* **154:**1092-1098

35. Nadziejko C, Finkelstein I, Balmes JR. (1995) Contribution of secretory leukocyte proteinase inhibitor to the antiprotease defense system of the peripheral lung: effect of ozone-induced acute inflammation. *Am Rev Respir Crit Care Med;* **152:**1592-1598

36. Roberts RM, Mathialagan N, Duffy JY, Smith GW. (1995) Regulation and regulatory role of proteinase inhibitors. *Crit. Rev. Euk. Gene Express.;* **5:**385-436

37. Finlay GA, Russell KJ, McMahon KJ, D'arcy EM, Masterson JB, Fitzgerald MX, O'Connor CM. (1997) Elevated levels of matrix metalloproteinases in bronchoalveolar lavage fluid of emphysematous patients. *Thorax;* **52:**502-506

38. D'Armiento J, Dalal SS, Okada Y, Berg RA, Chada K. (1992) Collagenase expression in the lungs of transgenic mice causes pulmonary emphysema. *Cell;* **71:**955-961

39. Selman M, Montano M, Ramos C, Vanda B, Becerril C, Delgado J, Sansores R, Barrios R, Pardo A. (1996) Tobacco smoke-induced lung emphysema in guinea pigs is associated with increased interstitial collagenase. *Am J Physiol;* **271:**L734-L743

40. Hautamaki RD, Kobayashi DK, Senior RM, Shapiro SD. (1997) Requirement for macrophage elastase for cigarette smoke-induced emphysema in mice. *Science;* **277:**2002-2004

41. Finlay GA, O'Driscoll LR, Russell KJ, D'Arcy EM, Masterson JB, Fitzgerald MX, O'Connor CM. (1997) Matrix metalloproteinase expression and production by alveolar macrophages in emphysema. *Am. J. Respir. Crit. Care Med.;* **156:**240-247

42. Ohnishi K, Takagi M, Kurokawa Y, Satomi S, Konttinen YT. (1998) Matrix metalloproteinase-mediated extracellular matrix protein degradation in human pulmonary emphysema. *Lab Invest;* **78:**1077-1087

43. Damianio VV, Tsang A, Kucich U, Abrams WR, Rosenbloom J, Kimbel P, Fallahnejad M, Weinbaum G. (1986) Immunolocalization of elastase in human emphysematous lungs. *J Clin Invest;* **78:**482-493

44. Fox B, Bull TB, Guz A, Harris E, Tetley TD. (1988) Is neutrophil elastase associated with elastic tissue in emphysema? *J Clin Pathol;* **41:**435

45. Morris SM, Stone PJ, Snider GL. (1993) Electron microscopic study of human lung tissue after in vitro exposure to elastase. *J Histochem Cytochem;* **41:**851-866

46. Tetley, T.D., Smith, S.F., Winning A.J., Foxall, J.M., Cooke, N.T., Burton, G.H., Harris, E. and Guz, A. (1989) The acute effect of cigarette smoking on the neutrophil elastase inhibitory capacity of peripheral lung lavage from asymptomatic volunteers. *Eur. Respir. J.* **2:** 802-810

47. Takeyabu K, Betsuyaku T, Nishimura M, Yoshioka A, Tanino M, Miyamoto K, Kawakami Y. (1998) Cysteine proteinases and cystatin C in bronchoalveolar lavage fluid from subjects with subclinical emphysema. *Eur Respir J;* **12:**1033-1039

48. Piccioni PD, Kramps JA, Rudolphus A, Bulgheroni A, Luisetti M. (1992) Proteinase/proteinase inhibitor imbalance in sputum sol phases from patients with chronic obstructive pulmonary disease. *Chest;* **102:**1470-1476

49. Vignola AM, Riccobono L, Mirabella A, Profita M, Chanez P, Bellia V, Mautino G, D'Accardi P, Bousquet J, Bonsignore G. (1998) Sputum metalloproteinase-9/tissue inhibitor of metalloproteinase-1 ratio correlates with airflow obstruction in asthma and chronic bronchitis. *Am. J. Respir. Crit. Care Med.;* **158:**1945-1950

50. Lee CT, Fein AM, Lippman M, Holtzman H, Kimbel P, Weinbaum G. (1981) Elastolytic activity in pulmonary lavage fluid from patients with respiratory distress syndrome. *N. Engl. J. Med. ;* **304:**192-196

51. Idell S, Kucich U, Fein A, Kueppers F, James HL, Walsh PN, Weinbaum G, Colman RW, Cohen AB. (1985) Neutrophil elastase-releasing factors in bronchoalveolar lavage from patients with adult respiratory distress syndrome. *Am Rev Respir Dis;* **132:**1098-1105

52. Christner P, Fein A, Goldberg S, Lippman M, Abrams W, Weinbaum G. (1985) Collagenase in the lower respiratory tract of patients with adult respiratory distress syndrome. *Am Rev Respir Dis;* **131:**690-695

53. Donnelly SC, MacGregor I, Zamani A, Gordon MWG, Robertson CE, Steedman DJ, Little K, Haslett C. (1995) Plasma elastase levels and the development of the adult respiratory distress syndrome. *Am. J. Respir. Crit. Care Med.;* **151:**1428-1433

54. Cochrane CG, Spragg RG, Revak SD. (1983) Pathogenesis of adult respiratory distress syndrome: evidence of oxidant activity in bronchoalveolar lavage fluid. *J Clin Invest;* **71:**754-761

55. Delclaux C, d'Ortho M-P, Delacourt C, Lebargy F, Brun-Buisson C, Brochard L, Lemaire F, Lafuma C, Harf A. (1997) Gelatinases in epithelial lining fluid of patients with adult respiratory distress syndrome. *Am J Physiol;* **272:**L155-L170

56. Bakowska J, Adamson IYR. (1998) Collagenase and gelatinase activities in bronchoalveolar lavage fluids during bleomycin-induced lung injury. *J Pathol*; **185:**319-323

57. Denholm EM, Rollins SM. (1993) Alveolar macrophage secretion of a 92kDa gelatinase in response to bleomycin. *Am J Physiol;* **265:**L581-L585

58. Swiderski RE, Dencoff JE, Floerchinger CS, Shapiro S, Hunninghake GW. (1998) Differential expression of extracellular matrix remodelling genes in a murine model of bleomycin-induced pulmonary fibrosis. *Am J Pathol;* **152:**821-828

59. Koslowski R, Knoch K-P, Wenzel K-W. (1998) Proteinases and proteinase inhibitors during the development of fibrosis in rat. *Clin. Chim. Acta;* **271:**45-56

60. Hayashi T, Stetler-Stevenson WG, Fleming MV, Fishback N, Koss MK, Liotta LA, Ferrans VJ, Travis WD. (1996) Immunohistochemical study of metalloproteinases and their tissue inhibitors in the lungs of patients with diffuse alveolar damage and idiopathic pulmonary fibrosis. *Am J Pathol;* **149:**1241-1256

Author Index